ONE WEEK LOAN

HYPNOTHERAPY
A Client-Centered Approach

HYPNOTHERAPY

A Client-Centered Approach

Mary Lee LaBay

Foreword by Patti McCormick

PELICAN PUBLISHING COMPANY
Gretna 2003

The word "Pelican" and the depiction of a pelican are trademarks
of Pelican Publishing Company, Inc., and are registered
in the U.S. Patent and Trademark Office.

Library of Congress Cataloging-in-Publication Data

LaBay, Mary Lee.
  Hypnotherapy : a client-centered approach / Mary Lee LaBay ; foreword
by Patti McCormick.
    p. cm.
Includes bibliographical references and index.
  ISBN 1-58980-052-4 (hbk. : alk. paper)
  1. Hypnotism—Therapeutic use. I. Title.
  RC495 .L25 2003
  615.8'512—dc21
                                                    2002008383

Printed in the United States of America

Published by Pelican Publishing Company, Inc.
1000 Burmaster Street, Gretna, Louisiana 70053

To my parents,
Maurice and Margery LaBay,
with love and appreciation

Acknowledgments

I give my heartfelt gratitude to my clients for the honor of facilitating and witnessing your healing and growth. I trust that our work together has enriched your lives as greatly as it has mine.

To my life partner, Scott: Your love and support have allowed me to realize my dreams in so many ways. I give you my love and appreciation.

I value the opportunities, encouragement, and assistance that I have received from Pelican Publishing Company. In particular, I would like to thank Dr. Milburn Calhoun, president and publisher; Nina Kooij, editor in chief; Kathleen Calhoun Nettleton, promotion director; Rachel Carner, promotion assistant; and Sally Boitnott, executive secretary.

Contents

Foreword

It is always with great pride that I watch a former student and now fellow colleague continue to move forward with their greatness. As I reviewed this manuscript, I became increasingly aware of how Mary Lee LaBay is truly following her journey of touching many lives with the power of knowledge. Her willingness to create a text that encompasses a self-directed approach to client care is a gift to the hypnotherapy profession.

As a registered nurse in the late 1970s, I worked in a cardiac unit of a major hospital. What that situation afforded me was the opportunity to compare a patient's clinical status with their emotional status. In many situations, I would see two patients who, in the nurse's station, looked identical. The blips on the cardiac monitor would be almost the same, and the laboratory results would match. As I would walk into each patient's room, I would many times see a totally different situation. Each patient's relationship with the disease process was entirely different, therefore greatly altering each experience of health. This would fortify my belief that a patient's attitude, family values, and general emotional state can greatly affect the outcome of an illness as well as continued quality of life.

We all experience this situation almost every day. Don't we all know a co-worker who has to take six weeks off for the "sniffles" while another co-worker goes to the opposite extreme and comes in to work with chest pain? Our attitude about health greatly affects our experience.

My curiosity about this phenomenon led me to search for ways in which we can affect the mind-body process. I was continuously looking for techniques to help patients learn how beliefs and past programming were influencing them. I also sought techniques that would help patients evaluate these core beliefs and change them if they so desired. My journey of exploration led me to learn of the clinical value of hypnotherapy.

Hypnotherapy is now recognized as a valuable tool that addresses the true components of mind-body healing. It also provides an opportunity for clients to create the change they desire and to discover the life they thought was only a fantasy. Research is continuing on the value of hypnotherapy in the medical and mental-health fields. According to a July 2001 feature article in *Scientific American,* the National Institutes of Health technology assessment panel judged hypnosis to be effective in alleviating pain from cancer and other chronic conditions. This article also stated that, in eighteen separate studies, patients who received cognitive behavior therapy plus hypnosis for disorders of obesity, insomnia, anxiety, and hypertension showed greater improvement than 70 percent of the patients who received psychotherapy alone. The American Psychological Association validated hypnosis as an adjunct procedure for the treatment of obesity.

With the increased substantiation of hypnotherapy's effectiveness, more highly trained hypnotherapy professionals are needed. Comprehensive texts such as this provide an excellent resource for individuals seeking training as well as current hypnotherapists seeking continuing education. Ms. LaBay's book presents solid hypnotherapeutic techniques from a client-centered perspective. When the hypnotherapist is wise enough to function from this parameter, client compliance increases tremendously.

I encourage everyone reading this text to be willing to explore the use of the techniques and concepts presented. Through them, they will find the core of mind-body-spirit healing.

Patti McCormick, R.N., Ph.D.
founder and president of Ohio Academy of Holistic Health, Inc.

Introduction

Hypnosis is an exciting field of study. Why? Because it provides us with tools to create change within ourselves, which, in turn, allows us to shape the lives that we choose to live. By altering our perceptions of the world, installing more resourceful behaviors, and aligning our emotional responses with the experiences that we have in the present, unencumbered by traumas of the past, we can become the masters of our own destinies. We can regain control of our lives. We can expect health and happiness and have viable techniques for achieving them.

We engage in a form of hypnosis daily, whether by choice or by default. We continually move in and out of our trance states about our identities and the reality of the world around us. What we consider our truth, or our reality, is simply a collection of ideas, perceptions, assumptions, expectations, and opinions that we have come to accept regarding the world around us and ourselves. Rarely are these estimations entirely accurate; generally, they are far from the truth.

It may be easier to recognize this as a fair statement if we turn our attention away from ourselves and look at the people around us. What do you notice about them? Ask yourself the following questions:

- Are they operating with clarity?
- Are they balanced?
- Do they function with a perfect view and understanding of the world around them?
- Are they free of habits, personality quirks, mood swings, or delusion?
- Do they exhibit full self-esteem?
- Are their reactions perfectly attuned to the events they experience?

• Are they aware of the unseen as well as the visible?

We could certainly generate more questions along this line. The point is, if we cannot find one person who can achieve a perfect and resounding "yes" response to all the above questions, chances are we, too, may fail on a few of those points.

In whatever area of our lives that we are not operating at the full glory and potential of our being, where our perceptions of our universe and of ourselves are skewed in some way, there we find the evidence of our trance states.

These may include negative self-talk, low self-opinions, hypocrisy, incongruity, violence, and self-destruction. These trance states may also include factors that may be considered positive attributes yet are equally removed from a balanced and clear connection with reality. Trance states may include altruism, a "Pollyanna" perspective, overconfidence, the schools of thought that expound such concepts as surrounding yourself in white light as protection from all evil, and so forth.

Mathematics principles teach us that A = A. Reality is only what it is—nothing more and nothing less. It just doesn't get any clearer than that. Any deviation from that axiom, in our perceptions, actions, and thoughts, constitutes a trance state.

You may be curious how we came to be so filled with illusion and delusion. Many factors contribute to our present mental, physical, emotional, and spiritual states. They may include a number of individual variations of a central theme: fear. There is fear of being:

• Different—That which makes you special makes you threatening to others. Being different frequently leads to being rejected, tortured, or killed. History is filled with horror stories of what has happened to people who tried the path of perfection. Furthermore, our personal histories include episodes of being teased, ridiculed, pointed at, and gossiped about, which support the terror of being different.

• Responsible—It has been said that with greatness comes responsibility. Many people find it uncomfortable to be culpable for themselves and those around them. Being responsible requires being conscientious and conscious, which, in turn, implies vision, decisions, and awareness of and accountability for consequences.

• Perfect—If we are to be perfect, we have no more excuses for shortcomings. There is a difference between a mistake and a sin. A mistake occurs when one did the best they could and the result was not as intended. A sin indicates that one knew better and proceeded anyway.

- Virtuous—When we see reality clearly, we cannot hide from our values. Being virtuous requires that we recognize our value system and then have the courage and conviction to uphold it.

We attain the above fears through subjective perspectives derived from:

- Conditioning
- Cultural norms, laws, and philosophy
- Religious teachings
- Life experiences
- Choice

Does this last one surprise you? We all have infinite choice. We can even acquire fear through a series of choices. So when clients come seeking assistance, they are exercising their choice to change whatever it is within them that no longer serves their life and ambitions.

A response I have been known to use when encountering those who justify things in their lives is: "How is it working for you so far?"

This question is meant to stimulate thinking outside the patterns and habits within which the person is circling. If a person continues to do the same thing over and over again, with the expectation that somehow the result will be different, perhaps they need to review basic principles of mathematics, which are an extension of logic, or vice versa. Remember A = A?

People come to practitioners of hypnotherapy in search of the catalyst to break their patterns. They seek the courage and conviction to overcome their fear and hesitation of fully regaining their true, powerful nature.

Through the techniques of hypnotherapy, rapid change can be attained. Encouragement, support, and movement along the path of healing and growth are, in themselves, further catalysts to continue the work. Many other, slower methods can lead to loss of faith in the possibility of attaining the goal. Disgruntled, bored, or financially and emotionally bankrupt men and women may lose the focus and energy to follow through with their objectives.

This book serves as a guide for that journey to attainment, whether the reader is anticipating taking up hypnotherapy as a career, adding it to their present work as a counselor or bodyworker, studying it out of curiosity, or desiring more knowledge for personal healing, growth, and path working.

As an introduction to the topic, it is well worth researching the colorful history of hypnosis, particularly in the context of the political and social settings of the day, to discover the legacy that has been given to us by many bright and bold forerunners.

Many indications of the use of trance are found in most indigenous cultural groups from ancient Egypt, to Greece, Africa, South America, the Pacific Islands, Asia, North America, and beyond. Trance states are associated with the works of medicine men, witch doctors, soothsayers, and religious orders. More recently, trance states have been associated with extraordinary feats of strength, with sports performance, and as alternatives to medical anesthesia.

Although mesmerism and hypnotism have frequently been linked, it may be surprising to learn that Anton Mesmer, in fact, did not intentionally use hypnosis, even though his experiments eventually led to the development of hypnosis and its applications. There were elements of hypnosis included in his methods, but these were not based on deliberate attempts or understanding.

Based on earlier writings that linked magnetism to the movements of planets, Mesmer (1734-1815) believed, as did others of his time, that he practiced an elaborate and unorthodox treatment of illness. His method was a system of smoke and mirrors. As we know, drama can play a profound role in the healing process, and drama was what Mesmer provided.

The stage for healing included a large tub (or *baquet*), which contained water, magnets, and iron filings. Patients would hold iron rods immersed in the tub. Sometimes the circle of patients grew so large that they would merely be touching each other or holding on to a rope that was reputed to connect them together. Mesmer would enter the scene dramatically, making "passes" in the air with his hands. Patients would have previously been instructed that these passes were supposed to direct to them a stream of the magnetic fluid from the tub. He would touch one of his patients, who would go into convulsions and then claim to be cured. Many subjects reported hallucinations, such as streams of dust or flames emanating from Dr. Mesmer's hands or from the magnets. It is no wonder that his greatest successes involved the remission of diseases considered hysterical in nature or origin. This is much the same way that cures are effected by faith healers. Notice the use of suggestibility, beliefs, drama, props, and the practitioner's confident attitude.

Mesmer's work received extensive criticism from the orthodox medical world in Vienna and Paris. He soon came under the investigation of a commission of inquiry ordered by King Louis XVI. The commission, whose president was Benjamin Franklin, included such well-known scientists as chemist Antoine Lavoisier (1743-94), who was beheaded by the guillotine, and the famous Dr. Joseph Guillotine. The commission carried on its investigation using the scientific methods available to it at that time.

It concluded that imagination without magnetism could still produce convulsions, and magnetism without imagination produced nothing. It was unanimously agreed that the magnetic fluid had no use whatsoever. In fact, it was determined that it did not exist.

Although the commission refuted any claims of success concerning Mesmer's magnets, their findings gave substantial support for the use of imagination in healing illnesses.

Although many believers in Mesmer's work continued their own experimentation, most documents erroneously attribute their success to magnets. In hindsight, we can see that the curative elements were more aligned with the techniques of modern-day hypnosis.

A contemporary of Mesmer, Fr. Joseph Gassner was a Catholic priest who created the trance phenomenon through religious ritual. Again, the drama combined with belief created substantial results. His place in history was assured when he created a trance so deep in a woman that two physicians pronounced her dead, whereupon he revived her.

Marquis Chastenet De Puysegur played his own small part in the history of hypnosis. As a student of Mesmer, he magnetized an elm tree in his hometown of Buzancy, France. Although misguided in his proposal to make diagnoses using extrasensory communication with the stomach, he is nevertheless credited with being the first person to induce somnambulism and to use hypnotic technique in the diagnosis of disease.

By the mid-1800s, Dr. James Esdaile published records of surgical operations in India using "mesmeric anesthesia." Other doctors and dentists were reporting similar successes. It is curious that the medical profession of that era received these studies with such ridicule and negation when, at that time, there was no chemical anesthesia available. Perhaps it has to do with the way that certain papers were written. There were exaggerated claims and lack of substantiation, perhaps creating more harm than support for the art.

James Braid, a Scottish doctor, coined the term "hypnosis" around the year 1842. Originally, the discipline was referred to as "neurypnology," meaning nervous sleep. His work was an attempt at making hypnosis respectable, bringing it out of the arena of assumptions, myths, and speculation that had been attributed to mesmerism.

In the latter part of the nineteenth century, Braid created an atmosphere for hypnosis to emerge as a reputable science. By carefully gaining the attention and respect of the medical community concerning this issue, he was able to step them through the logic and functioning of hypnosis. He replaced the word "mesmerism" with "hypnotism." His successes were based on his simple method of having his patients stare at a fixed point long enough to create eye fatigue. Although some of Braid's claims were not completely accurate, they also were not as absurd as those of the Mesmerists.

An important aspect was that he based his claims on the facts of anatomy and physiology known at the time. He brought to light the need in hypnosis for eye fatigue, willingness, and expectation.

Braid's work eventually came to the attention of Prof. Jean Martin Charcot, whose colleagues included Pierre Janet, Sigmund Freud, and Alfred Binet. Charcot noticed that hypnosis and hysteria shared many attributes. Later, Dr. Ivan Pavlov (1849-1936) would also use these studies for the basis of his experimentation. Charcot's theories would ultimately reveal half-truths and error. He held a fundamental belief that hypnosis could be produced mechanically, without the elements of expectation and suggestibility, elements that Braid's later findings determined to be critical. Further, he failed to experiment with hypnosis in normal people and thereby claimed erroneously that hypnosis could only be induced in those who were hysterical. He maintained that women were more susceptible to hypnosis than men were, basing that opinion on the traditional assumption that hysteria was the domain of women.

Meanwhile, two professors at the University of Nancy, Ambroise Liebault and Hippolite Bernheim, were developing this art along another path. They held that their subjects could go to sleep simply by the suggestion of the hypnotist. Their approach to hypnosis aligned with psychology as opposed to neurology and would eventually contribute greatly to the future of psychiatry. Liebault is considered by many to be the true "Father of Hypnosis," having recognized that hypnosis can be achieved by suggestion alone, without the added benefit of eye fatigue.

Charcot's pupil, Pierre Janet, furthered the intelligent use of hypnosis. He considered hypnosis to be a state of "dissociation"—a condition when one part of the mind operates independently from other parts. He found that information could be brought to light or be hidden from the conscious mind of his subjects. Repressed memories, for instance, could be regained. With an understanding of the times in which he was working, we can assume that many patients had not truly forgotten the information. Rather, out of shame or social convention, they may have simply refused, previously, to discuss these matters with their psychiatrists. Hypnotism may simply have served the purpose of allowing the subject to disclose information previously suppressed or secreted. At the same time, inexperienced hypnotists, along with devious or unwitting patients, were running the risk of creating false memories of experiences that never took place.

Along with Janet's theory of dissociation, which could be produced by hypnosis, or occur naturally during hysteria, there was the opportunity to study the phenomenon of multiple personalities and alternating personalities with "fugue states."

Although hypnosis inspired interest in these disorders, it was not to gain popularity at that time. In fact, over time interest in hypnosis waned, and it never really gained the respect from the medical community that it deserved. A small breakthrough occurred in 1892, when the British Medical Association's committee, which was appointed to investigate hypnosis, returned a favorable report. It stated that hypnosis was, in fact, helpful in inducing sleep, relieving pain, and alterating several functional disorders. They advised that only qualified medical personnel should facilitate hypnosis, and they further mandated that a female could only be hypnotized when accompanied by another female.

It is an interesting historical note that Sigmund Freud (1856-1939) studied under both Charcot and Bernheim and worked with Janet. He was well versed in the art and science of hypnosis as it was practiced in that day. Because at that time he was unable to determine in advance when a patient would prove to be a good hypnosis subject, he eventually chose to discard the entire field.

The difficulty may have rested in Freud's own personality, which may have railed against the idea of the occasional failure. Because hypnotherapy, as we know it today, is dependent on the willingness and susceptibility of the client, it is not necessarily the failure of the therapist when hypnosis is not achieved. Not understanding that, Freud went on to develop psychoanalysis, which had no implicit dangers of failure. Because psychoanalysts are enduring listeners, commentators, and interpreters of the words and experiences of their patients, there is no threat of failure to harm the therapists' reputations. Although psychoanalysis was an ingenious development, the method typically requires a longer path to recovery and change.

As it would happen, it would take the First World War to revive the need for and interest in hypnosis. The medical community would turn to hypnosis to treat the wounded and those suffering trauma-related illnesses. Freud's influence and the prestige of psychoanalysis would nevertheless continue to deny hypnosis's rightful place in medicine.

J. G. Watkins once again restored interest and prestige to hypnosis with his 1949 book entitled *Hypnotherapy of War Neuroses.* Using regression to cause an abreaction of traumatic emotions, he successfully relieved symptoms for veterans of the war.

Through his work during the middle of the twentieth century, Dr. Milton Erickson (1901-80) may have single-handedly legitimized hypnosis in the eyes of the medical community and brought it to the attention of the public at large. As a psychiatrist, he had the respect of the medical establishment. This was furthered by his unmatched genius and ability to create innovative strategies for healing and change in his patients. It was largely a result of his work that both the American Medical Association and the American Psychiatric Association at last endorsed hypnosis.

Highly respected Dave Elman (1900-1967) published the 1964 book *Hypnotherapy.* He contributed to hypnosis through his development of deep and rapid inductions and his indefatigable training of doctors and dentists in the techniques of hypnosis. Elman had an extraordinary life and made additional contributions to the American people that are worth further exploration.

Walter Sichort (1918-2000) was responsible for identifying and obtaining what he considered to be three depths of trance below somnambulism: coma, catatonic, and ultra depth. His colleagues have respectfully renamed the ultra-depth level the Sichort State.

John Grinder and Richard Bandler studied Milton Erickson and his techniques, which eventually led to their founding of the powerful field of Neuro-Linguistic Programming (NLP).

After many years of working together and writing books filled with their techniques and sessions, they have gone in separate career directions, continuing to produce leading-edge technology in this field.

An educator, publisher of works on hypnosis and hypnotherapy, and author of *Transforming Therapy: A New Approach to Hypnotherapy,* Gil Boyne is a political advocate who aids in the protection and validation of professional hypnotherapy.

Before his death, Charles Tebbetts was a revered hypnotherapist and trainer. Some refer to him as the "Grandfather of Modern Hypnosis." Tebbetts is the author of *Miracles on Demand: The Radical Short-Term Hypnotherapy.*

Author of *Hypnotism and Mysticism of India* and *Encyclopedia of Stage Hypnotism,* Ormond McGill is considered the "Dean of American Hypnotists." He has contributed decades of instruction, clinical work, and showmanship and has been a leader in combining Eastern philosophy with trance work.

Many other present-day practitioners are contributing new material or creating a change in the public attitude or political policymaking regarding the field of hypnotherapy. My own original contributions include the Reverse Metaphor and Empowerment Symbol, appearing here for the first time in a text.

By choosing to investigate hypnosis, the reader is entering a field of study with a colorful past. The people listed above all have made their contributions to the art, forming it into what it is today. Their body of knowledge, skills, research, and experience are the foundation upon which we, as practitioners, carry hypnosis into the future. It will be important to preserve the respectability of this healing art, while furthering its technology towards holistic complementary medical and spiritual capabilities.

The techniques and tools presented will allow the practitioner to address most all of life's issues. These may include a full range of physical healing, emotional rebalancing, mental clarity and training, and spiritual awareness and connection. The reason that these tools are so universal and potent is because they are based on the premise that, at some level, the clients or subjects are fully capable of determining their needs and the solutions for satisfying them. The level where this knowledge and wisdom can be accessed is frequently in the subconscious mind.

The subconscious mind, as implied in the name, is a subset of the human consciousness. The prefix "sub" signifies the consciousness that is below the surface. The subconscious mind has infinite ability to perceive and communicate at all levels. Incidentally, any use in this book of the term "unconscious" indicates being "not conscious," which occurs when one is passed out, in a coma state, out of body, or under chemical anesthesia.

Our presence in life is marked by two fundamental, irreplaceable factors: existence and consciousness. Our spirit is that which exists. Our consciousness is that which allows us to be aware that we exist. Life requires both. Life's purpose, at its most basic, is the maintenance, nurturing, and growth of our existence and consciousness. Lack of attention to this purpose will cause atrophy and perhaps eventual loss.

I join other practitioners in asserting that our physical, emotional, and mental bodies—their behaviors, perceptions, reactions, habits, symptoms, and more—provide concise and exquisite communications from our subconscious aspects. They inform us, whether by a whisper or a scream, of the needs required by our consciousness and existence and give indications of how and where we have strayed from the path of our soul.

The journey back to our connection and alignment with our essential nature is the goal of healing. Healing can take place through many methods. Hypnotherapy techniques are simply some of the options. They also happen to be viable, expeditious, and effective.

My personal journey began with an interest in philosophy, yoga, and meditation. Then, after years of pursuing avenues of personal growth and awareness, I decided to acquire a certification in clinical hypnotherapy. I chose the Ohio Academy of Holistic Health because of their extraordinarily comprehensive curriculum, which included psychology, anatomy, physiology, kinesiology, and more. They are now one of the only schools of this field that are federally accredited. Achieving my certification as a clinical hypnotherapist in 1997, I moved to the Seattle area and went on to become a certified NLP practitioner through Kevin Hogan (Hypnosis Research and Training Center) and Wil Horton (National Federation of NLP). In 1999, I received a Hypnotherapy Instructor's Certification through the Hypnosis Research and Training Center. During 2000, Kevin and I went on to write two books together. Along the way, I also received certifications as Practitioner of Reiki and Applied Kinesiology. What is presented here is a distillation of much of my training, combined with my personal and professional experience.

My work as a practitioner of hypnotherapy and NLP means more than a simple source of revenue, a career choice. Each of my clients brings a unique presence, quality, energy, and set of experiences into my life. It is fascinating to learn about each individual and their path, and it is powerfully satisfying to be a part of the process that allows them to make healthier and happier choices in their lives.

The present condition of one's life represents the culmination of all the choices one has ever made. Therefore, everyone is fully successful in this moment. Each of us has achieved exactly what we have worked towards throughout our life.

That can be a frightening statement if we are not ready to be responsible for ourselves. However, when one is prepared to be honest, the truth and wisdom in that statement will become apparent. Given the condition of some people's lives, this concept may seem harsh. Yet, within the responsibility exists the freedom to change. If we take responsibility for the present condition of our life, through the collective choices we have made, we can then take control of the choice to create a better life, as it is truly desired, through conscious awareness and selective experience.

Granted, some events appear to be out of our control. Yet, choice is still available. There is the choice to be a victim of circumstances or take an active role in overcoming obstacles, challenges, or setbacks.

Through these challenges, our morality—our virtues and values—is tested. Without choice there is no morality; without challenge there is no power; without struggle there is no self-esteem. Assist your clients in learning to embrace their trials. Victory is more than an easier life; it represents increased courage, conviction, and strength and is the evidence of self-love.

Recognition through rites of passage has always been an important step along the journey. These important ceremonies mark the initiation of the soul into higher levels of character. In their true essence, they are not given freely. They are awarded as a measure of a person's growth, through stringent trials. In many cultures, proof of strength, courage, valor, virtue, knowledge, or skill is required. When a person receives the rites, it is a prized representation of their new level of character, a new phase of their soul's growth.

In our modern society, we have all but lost our rites of passage. We graduate from high school or college and may not get another fragment of personal acknowledgment until the gold watch is received at the end of thirty years, simply marking the passage of time and representing the stamina of showing up every day for three decades. The human psyche needs more than that.

The human experience requires acknowledgment.

We require acknowledgment from others. We also require acknowledgment from ourselves. Although our parents may have led us to believe that we are lovable and worthy simply because we have been born into this world, as adults we come to realize that we need to earn respect, love, and self-love. Self-esteem cannot be given; it must be earned. How do we accomplish that? Self-esteem is earned by being righteous and victorious in our challenges.

My client files are filled with stories of challenges and victories. They are colorful stories of the making of private heroes. These are the people who love their life so much that they refuse to hide from it, suffer in it, or be a victim of it. They choose happiness. They choose to truly live.

My desire, in writing this book, is to offer tools that will aid many bright souls in their journey toward health and happiness.

My advice is to continuously pay attention to one's own healing and growth, humbly and honestly.

My promise is to do my part in aiding this healing and growth.

HYPNOTHERAPY
A Client-Centered Approach

PART I

The Clinical Practice

CHAPTER 1

Understanding Hypnosis

Controversy has surrounded the definition of hypnosis. Is it a state of mind? Is it a trance state? Is hypnosis a magical ability that a person develops to control another person?

This last question may have emerged from so many entertainers using "stage hypnosis" to get people to do outrageous things in front of an audience. Still, even in stage hypnosis the subjects are not really controlled. They are simply following the commands because there is a part of them that chooses to do so. This discussion will be left for another time. Let's just be clear that stage hypnosis is somewhat different from hypnotherapy, as practiced in the modern, holistic method.

Trance is an altered state of consciousness that occurs when we are not fully in the present moment, in mind, body, emotions, and spirit.

By this definition, it would seem that most people would have to declare themselves to be in a trance, or in hypnosis, most of the time! In fact, this may be true. It is curious how little time we spend really appreciating the present moment. Mentally, the human mind races from worries about the future to regrets concerning the past. Physically, our bodies demonstrate the sum total of our condition, as faithfully as would a history book. Emotionally, it is all too common to put away our feelings with the intent to deal with them at a more appropriate time. And spiritually—well, who really pays attention?

Therefore, we are all frequently in a state of trance. Our self-image, our levels of confidence, the "baggage" we drag around from the past, our recounting of our stories—all represent the trances we live in. It is most vividly shown when we drive past our exit on the highway, find ourselves daydreaming, or fail to catch what someone says because our "mind was somewhere else."

Beyond this more esoteric view of hypnosis and trance, there is the formal hypnotic state that a client enters when engaging in hypnotherapy techniques. For the sake of a common use of the term, we will define hypnosis as follows:

> **Hypnosis is the profound state of relaxation, focused mind, and heightened sensory awareness achieved when applied techniques take the brain waves of a subject to the level of alpha or below.**

Hypnotherapists Heal—Not Cure

To heal is to return to a state of health and wholeness. To cure means to remove the disease and its symptoms. Although these sound similar, there is a fundamental, and legal, issue at stake. The term "cure" is left to the medical community, their procedures, and their medications.

As hypnotherapists, we provide a space and deliver certain techniques that assist the client in changing and healing. The clients themselves are responsible for the results of the process. We cannot make them change or heal. We cannot guarantee results.

Hypnotherapists Cannot
Diagnose, Prescribe, or Evaluate

Unless you are a licensed medical doctor, refrain from giving your opinion on the labeling of symptoms, the cause, the solution, or the length of time it will take to heal. These activities are the domain of a licensed professional, whether medical doctor, psychologist, or other. Not only is it unethical to practice medicine without a license, or even practice hypnotherapy beyond your trained competence, the legal ramifications of diagnosing, prescribing, and evaluating are extensive.

When a client comes into the office with specific medical complaints, advise them to consult a qualified medical professional before commencing hypnotherapy treatments. If they already have, it would be prudent to contact that doctor and make sure that you are working in alignment with the medical treatment the client may be undergoing. It is crucial that the client seek a medical examination when they come to your office complaining of unexplained pain, migraines, or other symptoms, which could have serious medical implications. It could be life threatening to the client if pain were masked through hypnotherapy techniques, when it might be an indicator of a serious condition or disease.

Our bodies are equipped with the ability to give us pain as a warning that something is wrong. It serves a vital purpose. Once its purpose, its message, is delivered and is being acted upon, its severity can be diminished, through hypnotherapy or other means, for the comfort of the client.

Is Hypnotherapy a Tool of the Devil?

Let's address this issue right away. There are fearful people who would label anything unfamiliar to them as the work of the devil. You may come to your own conclusions based on experience and knowledge, rather than on speculation and rumor.

Imagine holding a knife. Is that knife the tool of the devil? We can determine that by asking what purposes it serves.

• Slice meat
• Cut wood
• Protect from harm
• Stab someone
• Open a box
• Substitute it for a screwdriver

Is the knife good or bad? It appears that it can save a life or take it away.

The answer is that the knife is neither good nor bad. The morality lies in the intention of the user. For any item you wonder about, simply put it through the same test. Certainly, you will come to the same conclusion. An item, or a technique, cannot be deemed good or evil, in and of itself. That is determined by the intentions of the individual wielding it.

So, are hypnosis and hypnotherapy good or evil? You are invited to put them through the test.

Self-Hypnosis, Autohypnosis, and Meditation

There are strong similarities between self-hypnosis, autohypnosis, and meditation. A simple explanation will lend clarity to their differences.

Self-hypnosis   Inducing hypnosis and administering self-help by using self-talk, chants, affirmations, and memorized scripts.

Autohypnosis   Same as above, since the prefix "auto" refers to "self" or "same." Popularly this term is used in reference to listening to prerecorded cassette tapes and compact disks.

Meditation   Passive observation of ideas and images and/or the clearing of the mind. Meditating does not popularly include the intent and plan for self-help or healing, though these may be by-products of the activity.

Techniques for Self-Hypnosis

Autohypnosis requires repetition to be effective. Although success can be achieved by listening to a guided visualization tape once or twice, results will be enhanced when this is practiced regularly over time. When using a tape that has been prerecorded, little preparation is needed. Simply find a quiet place, free of distractions, and settle in comfortably, whether sitting or lying down.

When preparing for self-hypnosis, without a recorded tape, it is wise to have written goals for the session. In a given session, optimal results will be achieved when only one or two of these objectives are addressed. It may also be helpful to have written suggestions or affirmations that can be read or recited during the session. Refer to chapter 18.

Keeping a notebook and pen handy is also practical. While you go into trance, you can deposit distracting thoughts on the paper for later consideration. Additionally, any breakthrough realizations, creative ideas, or helpful messages that are obtained can be recorded immediately so they are not soon forgotten.

When ready for the session, simply follow the above directions for locating a quiet place and relaxing comfortably. Staring at a candle, or at a spot on the wall at about a forty-five-degree angle upward, can aid in achieving trance. Both of these activities will create eye fatigue and flutters. When that occurs, simply close your eyes with the thought that doing so will take you deeper and deeper into trance.

Follow this with the Progressive Relaxation script in chapter 14, which is an easy one to memorize and administer to oneself. Use any desired visualization technique that encourages relaxation, release, and turning the attention inward.

Hypnosis—a State of Mind

We experience the trance state daily throughout our lives, whether by choice or by default. It allows us to respond automatically to stimuli and to take care of routine activities without constant attention and decision making. The intentional use of hypnosis techniques allows us to shape our lives, our responses, and our perceptions, creating the health and happiness we desire.

CHAPTER 2

Levels of Trance

In the previous chapter, the modern concept of trance was introduced. The following will give you an understanding of the traditionally accepted levels of trance as they pertain to the induction of formal hypnosis.

There is a controversy as to the number of levels of trance possible, and as to their descriptions and uses. Several detailed scales have been created, including:

- Davis-Husband Scale—Divides hypnosis into five major depths, with twenty-three separate levels.
- Cron-Bordeaux Scale—Displays six depths, with fifty indicators.
- Arons Six-Stage Scale—Describes six stages, with their correlating indicators.

Traditional Levels of Trance

Combining the various scales will produce a list similar to the following:

- Hypnoidal—Physical and mental relaxation; eye flutters
- Light trance—Catalepsy of small muscles; feelings of lightness or heaviness; will accept simple posthypnotic suggestions
- Medium trance—Catalepsy of large muscles; tactile, olfactory, and gustatory illusions; partial amnesia
- Deep trance—Somnambulism; complete amnesia; analgesia; positive hallucinations
- Deep somnambulism—Negative visual and auditory hallucinations; posthypnotic hallucinations, amnesia, and anesthesia

32

• Plenary trance—Stupor condition; no response to suggestions other than to move to higher levels

Recognition of Trance

There are various clues that will indicate to the hypnotherapist that trance is being achieved. Carefully observe your clients for the following overt indicators:

• Attentiveness—Are they focused on you, your words, or your actions? Are they undisturbed by minor distractions?
• Glazed eyes—If you are choosing eye fixation to initiate trance induction, it is typical to notice filminess over the eyes.
• Eye blinking—Once the filminess begins, the eyes will start to blink rapidly or "flutter."
• Eye movement—Once the eyes are closed, frequently there is rapid eye movement. On occasion, clients have commented that it is alarming or disturbing. If you notice it to be extreme, you may want to comment that eye movement and "fluttering" are normal indications of trance or hypnosis, so they feel assured.
• Bodily changes—You may notice in a client slower and rhythmic breathing and pulse rate, a change of color in the cheeks, and a change of skin temperature (if you should touch the client—which I rarely recommend).
• Swallow reflex—A client's swallow rate may decrease, unless a suggestion to the contrary is given for the sake of preventing dry mouth or proving suggestibility as in the Tasting Lemons test.
• Relaxation—This is particularly noticeable in clients who fidget and are restless during the intake interview and preliminary process of induction. Later in the session, you may begin to observe that they are fully relaxed and immobile. They may even state that they feel unable to move their arms or hands.
• Response to suggestions—These may include suggestibility tests or other observable movements.
• Reorientation—Upon emergence, the client may appear drowsy, move slowly, talk softly, or appear to have difficulty readjusting to the present time and place.

Besides the above observable indicators of trance, your clients may comment on the experience. They may describe the following:

- Visual alterations—If you are using an eye-fixation induction, the clients may notice their vision blurring, the object moving or appearing to vibrate, or changes in size or shape of the object or items in their peripheral vision.
- Sense of relaxation—Many clients state that they have never previously been so relaxed.
- Body sensations—Some clients experience their bodies melting into one with the environment or feel as if they are flattening or expanding. Their limbs may feel numb, cold, or warm.
- Enhanced or selective awareness—The client may experience an acute awareness of the surroundings as well as a "meta" awareness of their life, or they may narrow the focus of their attention to the exclusion of their surroundings and all but the nucleus of their session.
- Weight alterations—The body may feel heavier or lighter.
- Disorientation—Clients may temporarily be unaware of where they are or may experience events and memories in a dissociated state.
- Unexpected responses—They may comment that they were surprised to respond in a certain way to a suggestion. They may be surprised by emotional abreactions.
- Time distortion—Frequently clients will state that the session seemed to take only from half to a quarter of the time actually spent in trance. Alternatively, they may state that it felt they were in trance for a long, long time.

When you acknowledge their experiences, clients can trust that they have experienced trance, their reactions have been normal, and they can gain confidence in the successful outcome of their therapy.

Facts about the Trance State

In this trance state, anyone can be hypnotized. While everyone can, and frequently does, enter a hypnotic trance state, they remain capable of controlling their actions. No one will commit an act unless at some level they morally agree with it.

Any dangers in the use of hypnosis lie mostly in the ability of the hypnotherapist. Even with the best of intentions, when the techniques are not skillfully applied, or if the practitioner uses leading questions, implants improper suggestions, or in some other way abuses the client, there can be great danger.

A frequent question concerns whether a person could get lost in trance and not come back. There is no danger of clients failing to emerge from the hypnotic trance state. The worst that could happen is that they would fall asleep and awaken naturally sometime later.

The purpose of hypnosis is to allow our bodies to relax deeply and our minds to focus with clarity. It facilitates the ability to see life from a different perspective and receive information from our subconscious minds that may not have been readily available otherwise. Under hypnosis, we are more susceptible to accepting suggestions, which can lead to rapid changes in behavior and healing.

When the techniques are thoroughly studied and the hypnotherapist is vigilant in remaining client centered, nonleading, gentle, and compassionate, the work can be very powerful and safe.

CHAPTER 3

Imagination

One of the key ingredients of hypnosis and hypnotherapy is imagination.

Everyone uses imagination. It takes imagination to understand the spoken language. When a person says, "Put the coffee cup on the table," the listener has to imagine the message, and the requested act, before executing it. They have to imagine doing the task in order for their muscles to respond appropriately.

> **If you can imagine it, it can be made real.**

In hypnotherapy, sadly, we often find that our clients cannot imagine themselves in the state of health and happiness. They cannot imagine being prosperous, in loving relationships, successful, or thin. When they cannot imagine it, chances are it will never become a reality. The first effort of the hypnotherapist will be to help them learn to imagine their desires.

What we spend our days thinking about is what will become real for us. This is what will happen. It is not about magic. It is not ideological nonsense. It is easily demonstrated.

Our Mental Filters

When people are of the mindset that, say, everyone is out to cheat them, they will seek out substantiation of this. Their mental filters will spot every example of that "reality" or "truth," enlarging them and making them colorful and plentiful. All the experiences to the contrary will fall into a little-recognized mental file, small, pale, and insubstantial. Their philosophy will be vindicated and supported. If they cannot imagine a world where people can be trusted, it simply will not exist for them.

On the other hand, many of us know optimistic people, with bubbly accounts of the good and fortunate lives they lead. They exude happiness and good luck. Everything seems to turn out well for them and we wonder how they can do that.

These people live in the same world. They are exposed to the same nightly news and may have similar lifestyles. In fact, pairs of such people have been known to live in the same household! How is that possible?

It is all about perception. It is how they imagine their world to be, and therefore, it is.

Imagine the World You Desire

In our hypnotherapy practices, we must strive to assist our clients in enhancing the basic ability to be imaginative and, further, to adjust their filters to create the healthy, happy world they desire.

This is not to say that pain, disease, poverty, negativity, crime, and war are to be ignored. They, too, are a part of life. However, the goal is balance, along with hope, creativity, and the attainment of our dreams and purpose.

Steps to Enhancing Imagination

To increase imagination, it is important to use it. Stretch it. Expand it. Push at the edges. Imagination can be enhanced by:

• Reading books, especially science fiction and fantasy fiction
• Watching imaginative programs, especially science and science fiction
• Studying mathematics
• Enjoying or creating artwork
• Daydreaming
• Writing fictional stories
• Making up stories to tell to children
• Listening to creative visualization tapes and letting your imagination go wild
• Listing a number of outrageous and impractical solutions to problems
• Allowing yourself to mentally "dance" on the notes of music
• Engaging in free-flowing dance movements
• Practice, practice, practice

Cherish Your Imagination

Imagination is the wellspring of creativity. It is chaotic and unbounded in its natural state. It is the basic ingredient in the perception of reality. Everyone has the ability to imagine. It is a matter of how fertile or how constricted it is made to operate.

When the imagination is restricted, there are narrow margins defining life and its expression and experience. The broader and freer the imagination, the grander, more varied, and more infinite the experience of life.

CHAPTER 4

The Intake Interview

First Impressions

The interview actually starts the first time the client hears about the hypnotherapist. At that instant, they are forming an opinion about the hypnotherapist's character, qualifications, and skill level, plus the reputation implicitly or explicitly expressed by the source of their information. They may have seen an advertisement in a publication, read an article by or about the hypnotherapist, or come across a catalog of classes or workshops being presented. A direct referral may have been given by a colleague or satisfied client. Regardless of the source, opinions are forming about the level of trust, comfort, and rapport that may be expected.

Your Web Site Represents You

The potential client may turn to the Internet in search of a suitable therapist or for further information. The availability of a professional Web site not only lends credibility but gives the hypnotherapist a tremendous opportunity to:

- Reveal their background and training
- Explain their style and approach to the techniques
- Provide definitions and explanations of the process
- Give testimonials concerning their success
- Encourage the client to make an appointment or buy materials
- Link with other Web sites as a means of marketing and sharing information

Design your Web site in a manner that is inviting, easy to navigate, informative, and respectful.

What the Voice Reveals

The second phase of the interview occurs when the client and hypnotherapist speak on the telephone. The client will make their assessment of the hypnotherapist's character and ability by silently asking themselves the following questions:

- Is this hypnotherapist friendly?
- Do they seem to be knowledgeable?
- Do they make themselves available to explain and answer questions?
- Are their voice tone and attitude pleasant?
- Do they seem to embody compassion and empathy?
- Can they be trusted?

The hypnotherapist will be assessing whether to accept this new client by silently asking themselves the following questions:

- Am I qualified to assist this person?
- Is this person safe, or do they have ulterior motives?
- Will this person be financially and energetically committed to the process?

When speaking with potential clients on the phone for the first time, pay very close attention to the way that they express themselves. Are they clear about what they are seeking? Are they respectful about taking up time and energy? Do they truly want to heal or engage in self-discovery, or are they being pressured into it by a loved one? Do they give off the impression that they may not show up to their appointments?

A standard office policy may include a clause that appointment changes and cancellations must take place more than twenty-four hours in advance. A first-time client will not know this because they have not seen the disclosure statements. You may find that explaining the policy at the time the appointment is set, simply and respectfully, reminds them that this is a serious professional business and that everyone's time must be respected. No one should be offended that it is mentioned on the phone in advance. It will reduce "no-shows" to only those well-meaning folks who simply forgot or had a personal emergency.

The First Office Visit

The next, and most potent, time that an interview is taking place is actually in the office during the first appointment. This is a wonderful and fascinating opportunity to get to know another human being. It can be very special to connect with a person who has taken the time to seek you out, to ask assistance, and to commit to paying to receive the benefit of your skills and wisdom and who has arranged to show up in your office. You have to appreciate them!

During the intake interview, both the hypnotherapist and the client will have a very important opportunity to learn about one another. At this time, it will be mandatory to determine, with confidence, that the two parties are properly matched. This is when the most significant rapport building takes place.

In the rare case when one or both of the parties feel uncomfortable about working together, it is best to bring that to light as soon as possible.

If either of the people involved are not interested in furthering the client-therapist relationship, it must end immediately. The potential success of the session will be greatly diminished, if not eliminated. No one will benefit from continuing the session, and the reputation of the therapist, or the well-being of the client, is very much at risk.

In most cases, the parties are comfortable, and the task is to collect the information that will be vital to the session.

Required Forms

The first thing that must take place is the completion of the requisite forms. It is convenient to e-mail the forms to clients ahead of time so they can bring them to the office already completed. In this way, they will have the chance to read them over carefully and think about their answers and the topics they wish to cover in their session, and, of course, it saves time while they are in the office.

Client Intake Form

Consider including the following information on your intake form.

- Name
- Address
- Phone and e-mail
- Preferred time for follow-up calls
- Age and birthday
- Names and ages of people they reside with
- Marital status and number of children
- Occupation and place of business
- Who referred them
- Medical history, including doctors they are working with and medications they are taking
- A list of possible issues that may be addressed and therapy techniques available, with space for them to indicate which ones they are interested in
- Blank space for the client to add comments and concerns
- A statement regarding payment policies and payment methods accepted
- Any statements required by local governing bodies
- Signature and date line

The purposes of many of the items listed above are self-evident. By listing several different issues that can be addressed and therapy techniques available, people become aware of the possibility that healing can occur in areas or around subjects that they had not previously considered. Additionally, it may pique their curiosity about topics they may want to explore in the future.

Some hypnotherapists also request information concerning hobbies, number of siblings, birth order, spiritual practices, and deaths in the family in an effort to further understand the lifestyle of the client. In many locations, it is required by law to include certain information in the intake form. This may cover confidentiality, payment policies, and methods by which payment can be made.

The Disclosure Statement

The second necessary form is the Disclosure Statement. Again, the inclusion of certain information may be mandated by local governing bodies. These may include a registration number, education, training and background, methods of treatment, confidentiality and payment policies, and so forth.

Check with your local governing body for requirements in your area.

Enjoy the Interview

Beyond all the forms and regulations, remember that the primary purpose for the meeting with your client is to assist another human being in their quest for healing and change. Relax and enjoy the opportunity to make a difference in the world.

CHAPTER 5

The Office Atmosphere

The office setting will be an important aspect of your business. Although your clients primarily come to you because of your professional skills, they may not return if your location is not conducive to their relaxation, comfort, and trust. The three important elements to pay attention to in your office are the spatial, auditory, and olfactory environment that you have created.

The Spatial Environment

Providing a nurturing, clean, comfortable space in which to do your work is an important aspect of the overall healing. The client needs to feel safe and relaxed.

Imagine their experience. They are coming to a place they probably have never visited before. Perhaps they are meeting you for the first time. They anticipate being vulnerable. Their senses will be on high alert, determining whether they have made the right choice, they will be safe, and you can be trusted.

It may be prudent to remove signs of religious affiliation and cultural items that may taint sessions such as regression. Even family pictures may trigger negative emotions in someone who has just lost a loved one, has abandonment issues, or is in the midst of a divorce.

Walk through your space as though you were a stranger entering it for the first time. What do you notice? How does it feel? Is it clean, inviting, orderly, and esthetically pleasing? Does your space encourage relaxation and openness?

> **Treat your clients as though they were guests in your house.**

Consider providing your client with a reclining chair, several pillow choices, a blanket, an eye mask, and a glass of filtered water. Some people may use a few of the items, while others use none. However, the choices are available, and the clients will sense they are being cared for.

The Auditory Environment

The selection of music is another important atmospheric consideration. Gentle classical or New Age music can greet the client as they enter your office and during the intake process. The music chosen for the actual therapy session will have to be considered much more.

The selections most conducive to a nonleading, relaxing session include harmonious, measured, flowing music without very pronounced melodies. Avoid nature sounds, anything that even slightly indicates an ethnic origin, and anything fast paced or staccato.

Consider these titles for your collection:

- Psychosensory Integration Series, Programs 2 through 5, available through Brain/Mind Research, 204 N. El Camino Real, Suite E116, Encinitas, CA 92024. These can sometimes be ordered through your favorite music store. The intriguing aspect of these selections is that they include brain-wave synchronization technology.
- Dreamflight I, II, and III, the gentle, intuitive music of Herb Ernst. These CDs and more of his elegant productions are generally readily available at music and New Age retailers.

> **The healing qualities of music are vast.**

Be aware of how your clients are responding to the music that you choose for your office. You may even want to ask for their opinion. Whether or not you understand how to use music to your advantage, you certainly will not want it working against you in the healing process.

The Olfactory Environment

Soft, pleasant smells in the office atmosphere may enhance the comfort and ease of your session. You may want to learn about aromatherapy and the uses of specific aromas that facilitate the state you are aiming for.

Be aware, however, that many people have allergies to certain scents and chemicals in perfume, incense, oils, room fresheners, etc. Furthermore, certain perfumes or after-shave lotions may carry an anchor to a memory for the client that may be positive or negative.

> **Fresh neutral-smelling air is always a safe choice.**

If you are uncertain whether your office is inviting and comforting to your clients, consider asking the opinions of several close friends or colleagues. Many professional services are now available in most urban areas, such as feng shui consultants and clutter coaches. Attention to these details may prove to be critical in the building of your practice.

CHAPTER 6

Interviewing the Client

Once the hypnotherapist is in possession of the completed forms, the discussion can proceed. What will be interesting to find out will include:

- What brought them to the office today?

Realize that the issues that people are dealing with have typically been going on for some time. Frequently, the root cause of the issue lies far in the past. Aside from that, what was the event that finally triggered an appointment with a hypnotherapist?

- What are their goals for having hypnotherapy?

These will be indicated by the checkmarks that are next to the items on the intake form. However, further questions will be necessary to understand how these items affect them personally.

Helpful questions may include but are not limited to:

- Can you describe the pain that you mention?
- In what way do you experience blocks? How do they affect your life?
- What types of relationship issues do you have?
- What kinds of stress do you have in your life?
- How do you experience anxiety?
- What do you mean by work issues? What is happening there?
- Can you describe your health issues?
- How long have you been experiencing these symptoms?

Notice that these questions are nonleading. They simply are a request for more details to allow for a greater understanding of what is being presented.

Avoid Assumptions

It is vitally important that we do not assume to know what people are experiencing. We do not share their same set of experiences, knowledge, limitations, or perceptions. What is overwhelming to one person may be a minor irritation to someone else. Similarly, when it comes to pain, we have no way of knowing exactly what they mean. Do they mean physical, emotional, or mental pain? What are its qualities—sharp, dull, throbbing, etc.?

Ask questions. Get them to talk.

It could very well be that simply being able to express their condition and experience will play a major role in the healing process for a good number of your clients.

Many people have no one to talk to who will listen without judging, advising, mothering, abusing, dismissing, or ignoring them. There can be great relief in being allowed to freely share thoughts and emotions, reveal pain and fear, and disclose vulnerabilities.

Be a good listener. Nod. Smile. Look them in the eye. Be with them.

Confidentiality

Confidentiality is an issue regulated by the state concerning the therapy session. It can be much more extensive than you may have previously guessed. Confidentiality with your client means:

- Every piece of information exchanged between you, whether written or spoken, remains between only the two of you.
- The notes in your files must remain confidential.
- Your files concerning the case must stay in your sole possession, until which time it is legal for you to destroy them. Then they must be completely destroyed.
- The fact that a person is your client is confidential information. You cannot even initiate a conversation with that person in public. They must speak with you first if they choose to disclose that they know you.

Exceptions to the confidentiality guidelines include:

- If your client reveals a plan to commit a crime, it must be reported to the authorities.

- If your client is a minor child who reveals they have been abused, or who you suspect has been abused, you must report that to the proper authorities.
- If your files are subpoenaed by an authorized court of law, you must turn them over in accordance with your state or federal laws.
- When the client has requested that a third party be in the room, have them sign a waiver to that fact, explaining that anything that transpires during that time will not be protected under the usual confidentiality.
- Should your client request copies of your notes or request to record the session, have them sign a waiver that this has occurred and that you are no longer bound by the usual confidentiality.

Extracting Information

During the interview period, determine:

- The origin of the presenting issue. When did this condition begin?
- How do they know that it is an issue? How does it affect their life?
- Ownership. Is it the client's problem, or does it belong to someone else?
- Motivation. Are they in therapy for their own reasons or at the urging of another person?
- What is the client's expectation of the session?
- What is the client's perception of the cause of the issue? What is behind it and what do they feel would change or remove it?
- Decide on reasonable goals for the session together.

Who Is in Control of the Session?

It is common for a client to expect a hypnotherapy session to resemble a stage hypnosis. This is understandable, since most people have only been exposed to the concept of hypnosis through television, movies, and, perhaps, live stage shows.

In fact, hypnotherapy is quite different. It is different in intent and technique, as well as in results.

In stage hypnosis, the intent is to entertain. A large number of people are given certain suggestibility tests in order to discover who would be the best subjects for the show. These candidates are then led through two or more further tests to eliminate all but the most cooperative and susceptible subjects. These subjects are highly imaginative, are willing, and have the desire to experience this phenomenon.

This gives the audience the impression that the powers of hypnosis are great and far reaching and that the hypnotist has supernatural control over the subjects. In reality, those people who were not cooperative were simply removed from the demonstration.

The intent of hypnotherapy, however, is to discover the motivations and intentions of the subject and to facilitate change for their greater health and happiness. During a typical session, the will and desire of the client is of foremost importance. They will be able to determine the speed and direction of the session.

Length of Interview

The time that it will take to discover the necessary information will depend on the client and the issues presented. Some hypnotherapists take the entire first session to discuss the issues and an appropriate plan for future sessions. Another approach would be to collect a suitable amount of vital information and then continue the discovery while the client is experiencing trance. Over time, you will develop a comfortable feel for the necessary length of of an interview.

CHAPTER 7

Ingredients of
Successful Hypnotherapy

Many individuals shy away from hypnotherapy, fearing they would not be able to let go and be hypnotized. They think that it would involve giving up their control. It is beneficial to explain to such individuals that during the session they are always in control.

- They will be aware of the fact that they are in dialogue with the hypnotherapist.
- They are free to open their eyes, refuse to answer questions, indicate their desire to move the session in a

> **Success will be enhanced when the subject brings cooperation, desire, and positive belief into the session.**

different direction, or proceed at a different pace.
- If they need to use the restroom, want a glass of water, or prefer to change the temperature in the room, they simply have to express that.

When assured that they will be control—or at least not "out of control"—most clients feel safe enough to proceed. If the client still experiences some hesitation, it would be wise to begin the session with that very issue.

Such a quandary would make a perfect Parts Therapy issue, a technique that will be presented in a later chapter. Part of the client wants to go into hypnotherapy, or they wouldn't be in your office, and part of them is resisting, or fearful of that. Start there, and when that issue is resolved, the client will already be in trance, and any blocks to proceeding should be removed.

Only the client can allow hypnosis to take place. Feel free to inform them of that. It gives them the rightful responsibility for the success of their trance level and assures them that you are not doing anything to them. They are doing it for themselves.

The session is about the client, not about the therapist.

Rapport between the Client and the Therapist

Rapport is a sympathetic and harmonious relationship. This is a vital ingredient in the successful hypnotherapy session, because without rapport there will be tension and discord, whether subtle or tangible.

Rapport building begins with that first contact and continues with each interaction of the two parties. Because the sessions are client centered, it is the responsibility of the therapist to adjust into rapport with the client.

If the hypnotherapist is simply unable, or unwilling, to fine-tune themselves in accordance with the client, it may be best to refer the client to another hypnotherapist. Reasons why this may occur could vary from discomfort with the subject matter disclosed to a distinct discord of styles, personalities, or morals.

Many tactics can be utilized to build rapport. Here is a sampling of skills that can be practiced both in the clinical setting as well as in relationships in one's personal life.

Mirroring

Practice subtly mimicking the bodily positions exhibited by the other person. When they sit forward, move forward. When they cross their arms or legs, follow suit, subtly and apparently unconsciously.

Eye Contact

Look the other person in the eyes, holding attention on them, without simply staring. This may involve tilting your head to one side, nodding faintly from time to time, and exuding a sense of sympathy, agreement, or understanding.

Eye Alignment

The majority of people will report that they feel more positive about the person in front of them when their right eyes are making the dominant

> **Experiment: Sit facing a person slightly off to their left, so that your left knees are aligned (not touching, of course) and your left eyes make the dominant contact. Converse for a few moments and notice how you feel emotionally and energetically.**
>
> **Now shift your position slightly so that your right knees face each other and your right eyes make the dominant contact. Observe your feelings and reactions this time.**

connection. You may find it amusing to realize this is how we greet people when we shake hands. It is a fortuitous custom.

With this in mind, pay attention to the configuration of furniture in your office. How the chairs are placed will affect which eyes are connecting.

Verbal Agreement

You may or may not be totally in accord with the opinions and perspectives of another person. However, you may find it possible to enhance the rapport between you, even while silently disagreeing, if you use a few simple phrases. These may include:

- "I see what you mean."
- "I understand."
- "I can sympathize with you."

None of these statements indicates that you agree with their perspective or philosophy, yet they lend support to that person's experience and emotions.

Breathing

A very subtle and powerful method of gaining rapport is to breathe with the other person. Watch for the rising and falling of their chest and stomach, and match your breathing accordingly. Inhale and exhale at the same time, and at the same pace, with them.

Energy

This is an area of rapport frequently overlooked, yet extremely important. Try imagining a cocoon of positive, white or pastel energy surrounding your office. That alone may shift the feelings experienced in this encounter.

> **Experiment: With three people participating, assign one person to be the client and ask them to leave the room so they don't hear the following instructions. Of the two remaining participants, one will be designated as the counselor and the other as the observer. The counselor will ask questions of the client while thinking positive thoughts and exuding supportive, loving energy to that person. When the observer gives a cough, the counselor continues with the questioning but now thinking negative thoughts about the client and exuding negative energy. Do this without changing facial expressions or body posture. It is a change in thought and energy only. The observer will give another cough and the counselor will return to positive thoughts and energy. Throughout the exercise, the observer will be noticing any changes in the client. Watch for signs in the client of: open/closed, comfort/ discomfort, and upbeat/depressed, plus changes in body language, posture, speech patterns, and so forth.**

It is typical to notice overt signs of change in the client's attitude and connection with the therapist, solely based on the energy that they are receiving. Learning to manipulate your energy to gain more positive results with your client (and your friends and family) will be a valuable skill throughout your life.

Therapeutic Alliance

Therapeutic alliance means that you are on the same team, working in synchronization with the client towards a common goal. The goal in this case is the healing of the client. Their best interest is at the center of the session.

It is possible to achieve and maintain that alliance by staying focused on the highest and best outcome for the client. Ask questions that allow you to understand their goals, both short and long term. Find out what they want to achieve through hypnotherapy overall and then narrow the focus, asking them what it is that they would like to take away from the present session.

Ask the client to prioritize their list of goals. What is the most important item they would like to address first? Then, what would be next?

Naturally, it is expected that the therapist will learn not only everything about what the client indicates they are experiencing, but also whatever can be gained from other resources about the issues presented, and all the possible therapy techniques that are advisable in this case.

Let the client know, with certainty, that you are working together for the best outcome of the situation.

Transference

Transference in the clinical context means that the client has substituted the hypnotherapist for someone else in their life. Transference can work for the hypnotherapist and against them.

In the negative context of transference, the client may confuse the blame or anger they feel regarding another person and turn it against the hypnotherapist. Likewise, transference may occur if a lonely client turns their affection from a lost loved one to the hypnotherapist.

These are not healthy situations and must be remedied promptly. Immediate conversations to straighten out the issues must be initiated. Clarity must be obtained. If that does not appear to be possible, it is advisable to refer that client to another therapist.

On the positive side of transference, the client may find that they can borrow the therapist's sense of confidence, security, or balance while they are regaining and strengthening their own. Although the sights must be set on the client's own ability to obtain these qualities, this can be a supportive intermediary step.

Countertransference

When countertransference occurs, the therapist is internalizing or identifying with the information given by the client. When the hypnotherapist reacts emotionally to the information, or is distracted by it in such a way that a clear and client-centered session is not possible, the hypnotherapist needs to seek counsel of their own, and quite possibly it will be necessary to refer the client to another therapist.

Boundaries

This leads us to consider boundaries. This subject is not only a moral issue but a legal one. You must become very familiar with the legal regulations governing your practice in your own state. Most states have a two-year rule. This means there can be no gifts, lunches, dating, or sex between the parties for two years after the last professional session.

It is inappropriate, at the very least, to facilitate therapeutic techniques with close friends and relatives. It clouds the nature of the relationship, creates trust issues that should not be a concern within a healthy client/hypnotherapist alliance, and could ultimately damage the close personal nature of your relationship.

If you are simply facilitating stress reduction or providing guided visualization, it should not be a problem. It becomes risky when it moves toward delivering therapy.

It will be vital to have boundaries concerning your time as well as your space. This will proceed through issues of scheduling, days off, pricing, length of phone calls, personal relationships, ending the session, no-shows, and much more.

Be clear regarding boundaries. Learn to have good ones. Your clients will call on you frequently to help them with their own boundaries. Everyone will benefit greatly if you can serve as a good example of this issue.

Abreaction

An abreaction is the release of any emotion, due to the recall of a memory, the telling of a story, or other mental activity, such as imagination, metaphor, etc. Although it may take many forms, such as screaming or laughing, most typically it is expressed by tears, crying, or sobbing. Yet, not all clients cry, nor should they.

When they do, there is no need to worry. These emotions indicate that the hypnotherapist is reaching an area or subject that needs attention. These emotions may have been locked away for a long time, left to fester and create imbalance, illness, or dysfunction. Occasionally, a client claims that they will cry at anything. The release is still a positive step. Hand the client a tissue and encourage them to stay in touch with these emotions, feeling them, understanding them, and allowing them to be expressed.

Should a client articulate embarrassment about the tears, try to relax them by saying, in a gentle way, that abreactions indicate breakthroughs on the path to healing. In this way, they are encouraged to feel positively about their tears, as though they have achieved a milestone in their therapy—as they have!

Calming Extreme Abreactions

It occasionally occurs that a client begins sobbing and cannot regain composure. It goes on and on, until they are distraught. There is a handy procedure you can administer that actually belongs to the field of applied kinesiology.

Ask the client whether you have permission to touch their forehead. Wait for their approval. Request that they become fully engaged with the emotion. When they are feeling their pain, anger, outrage, guilt, etc., on all levels, ask them to rate the intensity on a scale from one to ten, with ten being the most intense. Then, gently apply your fingers to the "corners" of their forehead. The corners are the areas where the front of the forehead curve to form the top and sides. While holding your hands in this position, gently stretch the skin outward and hold. Do not rub, move your hands, stroke, or any such thing. Just hold your hands still, pulling slightly.

This is a natural place where people touch themselves when they receive shocking news. Their hands immediately go up to their foreheads when they are deeply upset. Perhaps you remember your mother holding your forehead like that when you weren't feeling well as a child. Now you understand the healing properties of that touch.

Continue holding this position for your client until the emotions subside. You may notice them relaxing and letting out a deep sigh. They may say to you that they are having difficulty focusing on the problem anymore.

Ask them to again rate the intensity of the emotion. Expect the reduction in intensity to be significant, dropping from an original designation of eight to ten, down to between one and three. Ask whether that is a comfortable level for them. If it is not, continue with the procedure until it reaches the desired level.

Upon completion of this exercise, chat with the client about a nonrelated topic. Engage in a social conversation. This is called breaking state. It takes their mind off that immediate subject. Then, come back to the issue at hand, and ask them how they are feeling about it. This is called an environment check. We are determining the level of impact this issue still has for the client. They should respond that it is still at the lower level reached during the exercise.

The fascinating aspect of this procedure is that the emotions around the issue addressed will never return to the original level of intensity.

Caution: Only use the above technique for unwanted, negative emotions. We do not want to remove enthusiasm, joy, or love!

Abreactions are a healthy part of the therapeutic process. Emotions must be expressed. When bottled up, or left unacknowledged, they will manifest in other ways. They may erupt as rage, depression, weight gain or loss, weeping, nervous ticks, addictions, and chronic pain and illness, among many other dysfunctions and disorders.

One of the ultimate goals of the healing process is to regain the natural flow of appropriate emotional responses tied to immediate events. This translates into being in the present moment and responding to current happenings, in a clear and suitable manner.

Successful Results

By practicing the above techniques for building rapport and trust, creating boundaries, and handling abreactions, the client-hypnotherapist relationship will have a legal, ethical, and personally comfortable structure within which to flourish.

CHAPTER 8

Therapeutic Communication

Communication Style

Second only to the techniques that you use in your sessions, your voice is a primary force in the therapy process. Practice making it smooth, deep, resonant, and rich. This does not mean that it has to be loud. Rather, it can be gentle, soft, nurturing, and seductive.

Try matching your volume to the volume that the client is using. As they go deeper into trance, they will typically speak more and more softly. You may find yourself even whispering in conjunction with them. Imagine how jarring it would be to be totally relaxed and whispering, when another person in the room is speaking in a loud, booming voice! This is far from being in rapport.

Another point of pacing with the client is the tempo at which you speak. Again, if they are speaking slowly, you will want to match that. Imagine how it is when you are taking a nap or are extremely sleepy, and someone comes in the room speaking loudly and rapidly. It is most irritating! Please demonstrate empathy and rapport with your voice at all times.

Silence and Listening

One of the most powerful resources you have as a hypnotherapist is your ability to be in silence with your client. It may also be one of the hardest to learn and practice!

Patiently allowing clients to express themselves is very respectful and nurturing. It may be that they rarely get that opportunity in their daily lives. The majority of your clients are not coming to you for your words; they are coming to experience your silence.

How do you feel when you are distraught and pouring out your soul, only to be met with:

- Advice
- Mothering
- Criticism
- Scolding
- A bigger fish tale
- "I told you so"
- Shock and disgust
- Anger
- Sadness
- Shame
- Embarrassment
- Disappointment

Would you not long for someone who would just let you express yourself and would refrain from fixing your problems? Would you seek someone who would not insist on finding the answers for you?

Your clients come to you so that they can discover their own answers. Encouraging clients to connect with their own wisdom and strength will result in higher self-esteem, clarity, and rapid integration of the resolution.

Be silent. Listen. When you are quiet, the client will tell you exactly what is wrong and will discover a proper path to resolution.

Basic Rules for Communication

- Check yourself. Where are you mentally? Are you having a bad day? Are you feeling centered? Take the time to assess your own moods and thoughts. We all filter every experience through our own colored glasses. To the degree that they are layered with many personal issues and unresolved emotions and thoughts, our filters will cause us to receive communications, whether verbal or visual, in a manner that is distorted.
- Inquire into the meaning of the client's statements. Ask them, "What does that mean to you?" "What would I be experiencing if I had your exact symptoms?" "If I were to playact you in those emotions, what would I be doing?"

• Pay attention to what the client doesn't tell you. Even an offhand remark can indicate the true nature of the problem they are experiencing.

Staying Client Centered

At all times, and particularly within the clinical session, it is the responsibility of the hypnotherapist to remain "client centered." What exactly does that mean?

It is important to remember that when a client comes to see a hypnotherapist—or any therapist, for that matter—it is for the benefit of the client. It is their session. All too frequently, therapists find themselves interjecting their own philosophy, standards, beliefs, desires, needs, or dysfunctions into the session. This possibility can emerge quite inconspicuously and unconsciously.

The easiest way to remain client centered during the interview or in hypnosis is to stay very close to the following questions:

• What do (did you) you notice?
• What do (did you) you experience?
• What do you observe?
• What happens next?
• And then what?
• Where would you like to go?
• What would you like to do about that?
• How does that make you feel?
• Is there anything more?
• When did that occur?
• When will you be able to do that?
• What outcome would you like to have?
• Is there anything more you would like to do concerning this issue?

Granted, the types of questions will change somewhat when using advanced techniques discussed later in this book. However, these questions do provide insight into how to remain impartial, avoid leading questions, and maintain a clean, client-centered session.

Leading Questions

Leading questions might include:

• Are you referring to your father?

- Is that building a house or a barn?
- Are you sad to learn that?
- Was that a shocking experience for you?
- Did that occur when you were two or three years old?
- Will you be able to do that within the week?
- Would you like that to go away?

The list could go on indefinitely. You are surely getting the idea.

False Memories

Leading questions can give rise to numerous problems. One of the most controversial is implanting false memories. There have been many stories and articles in the media about the very real problem of false memories.

Since most of our memories are simply our perceptions and impressions of what we think is real, or what we think occurred, there is a school of thought that all memory is false memory. On the other end of the balance are those who hold that if you think it is real then it is real for you. Without debating this subject here, be mindful that the role of a hypnotherapist is to provide the space, energy, and techniques to facilitate the healing and changes desired by the client.

If a client discloses that they are seeking to discover forgotten memories with the intention of confronting or suing another individual or group for some offense, it is recommended that this client be referred to a qualified forensic hypnotherapist.

It is valuable for all therapists, including hypnotherapists, to regularly get help for themselves. We all need to have work done, improvements made, and our burdens relieved. Be sure to take care of yourself as well as you care for those who seek your help. When the hypnotherapist's needs are satisfied, there will be less chance of hidden personal agendas within the client's session.

The more balanced we are in our own lives, the greater clarity we bring to the hypnotherapy session for our clients.

Anchoring for Rapport

Anchoring is similar to Pavlov's stimulus/response. Everything that we do or experience sets up anchors. A good example of an anchor is an old tune that conjures memories of some long-ago event or relationship. That music anchors this present moment to that long-ago era.

We will discuss anchors as therapy techniques later in this book. We are discussing them here as techniques to be used advantageously in building and maintaining rapport.

- If you compliment your client while touching their elbow as they enter your office, you have set up a positive anchor to their good feeling about that comment.
- Once your client has had a satisfying and pleasant experience while in the chair in your office, it will be easy for them to slip into those good feelings once again when entering your office and sitting in the same chair.
- The use of the same music may make it easy for them to settle into trance, having anchored it to that state in previous sessions.

Even posture may anchor a mood. Notice how it feels to slouch and droop the head. Then stand straight and tall, with head uplifted. Notice the difference that it makes in your emotional state.

Your voice is a powerful anchor, especially when the client's eyes are closed. This can be enhanced through tone, speed, and volume.

> **Clients comment that, after having been in trance so frequently in my office, listening to me speak—whether in conversation or in a class—now creates an altered state for them.**

CHAPTER 9

What Clients Communicate

Our clients communicate to us in a number of ways beyond the words that they say. Actions, behaviors, postures, gestures, body language, symptoms, and incongruence are a few indications of what our clients may not be verbalizing.

Accessing Cues

Each one of us makes contact with the world we live in through our senses—sight, hearing, touch, taste, and smell. This information is stored in and retrieved from certain distinct areas of our visual range. These areas relate to the sense operating at the time of the experience. It is more easily understood by viewing the following diagram.

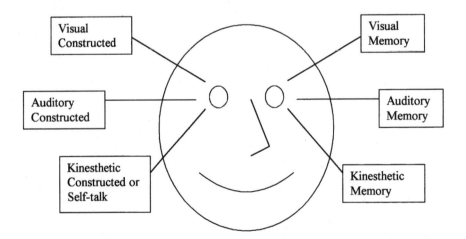

The diagram indicates that when a person is speaking about an event that they remember, they may look up to the left if they have a vision of this memory, look directly left towards their ear if they heard the information, or look down to the left if they remember the event through feelings.

If the person is telling a story that they have created, they will look right and up, directly right, or down, depending on whether they are imagining it visually, through sound, or as self-talk.

A small percent of the population will demonstrate a reversal of the left and right accessing. It is important to test the subject several times with information that you know to be memory based or constructed to confirm their accessing method.

Determine What Is Normal

To test for accessing cues, ask questions such as:

• What color are your spouse's eyes? (Remembered)
• What happened during your day at the spa? (Remembered)
• How would you look if you had bright blue hair? (Constructed)
• If you had a billion dollars, what would you like to do? (Constructed)
• What do you think it would be like to be the opposite sex? (Constructed)
• What did you do on your last birthday? (Remembered)

The preceding questions will help you to distinguish their direction for remembered and constructed thoughts. Then it is just a matter of observing whether they are looking up, to the side, or down, to determine whether these particular memories are retained through visual, auditory, or kinesthetic references.

How Can This Help the Hypnotherapist?

Knowing the eye accessing cues for your client may help you in two ways. If you are hypnotizing them in order to get details of an accident, you will want to determine whether they are really remembering an incident or whether they are fabricating or imagining these facts. It is also helpful to discern the difference when you have asked them to create a metaphor and you discover they are retelling an event that actually happened.

The primary use of the eye accessing cues, however, is to gain even greater rapport with the client. Adjusting your language patterns to match their experience will allow you to connect even more deeply with your client.

Clues for the Cues

The following words and phrases match the respective sensory channels:

- Visual—see, view, look, visualize, reveal, clear, brighten, dim, foggy, watch, appear, picture, sight, pretty, ugly, etc.
- Visual phrases—I see what you mean, picture this, short sighted, catch a glimpse, point of view, shed light on, picture perfect, etc.
- Auditory—hear, listen, sound, harmonious, deafening, tone, resonance, discordance, thunderous, buzz, chattering, loud, liar, crackle, etc.
- Auditory phrases—I hear you, listen up, describe in detail, tell the truth, hum a tune, sing a song, voice an opinion, fast talker, manner of speaking, I'm telling you, etc.
- Kinesthetic—feel, touch, cold, warm, hard, soft, grab, catch, rough, slick, slippery, wet, slimy, fluffy, velvety, thick, etc.
- Kinesthetic phrases—get in touch with, hot head, was touched, feel for you, warm hearted, handling it, firmly rooted, on solid ground, fell through, put it down, on the record, etc.

Additionally, words that relate to olfactory and gustatory senses, which are not accounted for in the diagram, include: sweet, sour, fishy, this smells of, stinks, rotten, spicy, etc.

Gestures

Beyond the eye accessing cues used for distinguishing the sensory correlations to memories, there are other gestures and habits.

People who are predominately visual may exhibit shallow breathing and higher-pitched voices and be expressive with their eyes, such as squinting, winking, etc. They tend to speak rapidly and use hand gestures above, around, and pointing to their eyes.

Individuals who tend towards auditory access may have fluctuating voice tones and knitted eyebrows and may turn their heads so their ears are forward when listening. Their hand gestures touch or point around and towards the ears, mouth, and chin.

Kinesthetic individuals show deeper abdominal breathing, deep sensual voice tones, and slower speech. You may notice them touching their chests and stomachs. Hand gestures are below the waist.

It is amusing to observe these accessing cues in conversations, both in the office and in the world at large. It broadens your knowledge about the experience others are having and allows you to create greater connections with them.

Leakage

Leakage refers to the unconscious nervous energy that shakes out of the ends of the feet and hands when a person is uncomfortable about the topic being discussed. Sometimes people are observed playing with their hair, fingers, fingernails, face, or clothing, or they tap their fingers, jiggle their knees, or fidget in some way.

A client was discussing her presenting issues, and as soon as the topic of her father came up, her feet started jiggling. Although she claimed there was nothing unusual about her relationship with her father, on closer examination, a childhood issue was discovered that needed to be addressed.

Understand What They Don't Tell You

You will find that your clients will use distortion, deletion, and generalizations in constructing their "reality." It is important to be aware of these and be able to respond appropriately when they arise. You may find that while speaking with your clients to clarify a distortion, deletion, or generalization, they will achieve tremendous breakthroughs in their issues.

Distortion

The use of linguistic distortion occurs in a variety of ways, in most of what we think and say, every day.

Mind Reading

> **Be vigilant of the "colored glasses" through which a person sees their reality.**

It is tempting to want to know what other people are thinking. In fact, some people think that they do that fairly well. Unless you are a professional psychic with the proven accomplishment of successful telepathic connections, it is best to stay away from trying to read people's minds. We are generally less accurate than we care to admit.

Fooling ourselves into thinking that we can read someone else's mind is a form of trance—a false reality—that we, and our clients, create. Learning to correct it in yourself will enhance your ability to assist your clients.

Ask questions. Following are statements and possible responses you can practice in your communications.

Statement: "They don't like me."
Response: "Who doesn't like you?" "What don't they like about you?"

Statement: "It hurt me."
Response: "In what way are you hurt?" "What is that experience like for you?"

Lost Subject

These statements of reality, or judgments, are made without stating the source.

Statement: "It is wrong to swear."
Response: "According to whom?" "Who says so?" "How do you know that?"

Cause and Effect Relationship

It is important not only to identify another person's perspective of the cause and effect in an event or situation but also to explore the person's responsibility for their perspective and response.

Statement: "He makes me mad."
Response: "What is it that he does, specifically, that makes you choose to be mad?"

Statement: "Rush-hour traffic really makes me angry."
Response: "What is it about rush-hour traffic that causes you to choose to respond with anger?"

This manner of constructing responses will demonstrate that the person is in control of their responses, reactions, and choices of how they wish to spend their lives. It returns responsibility and power to the person.

Complex Equivalence

This type of distortion draws conclusions that do not necessarily have a cause and effect relationship, and involves mind reading as well.

Statement: "My dad divorced my mom, and he left us. He doesn't love me."
Response: "How does your dad divorcing your mom mean that he doesn't love you?"

Statement: "Whenever he sees me, he looks away. He doesn't like me."
Response: "How does looking away mean that he doesn't like you?"
"Have you ever looked away from someone whom you liked?"
"Could there be other reasons why people look away?"

By exploring additional possible interpretations, the person has the opportunity to begin examining alternative perceptions, breaking out of the fixation of thinking that their interpretation is the only possibility.

Presuppositions

These are the axioms, the basic "laws of reality," that we form and hold to. From these we make unquestioned judgments about our experience. Typically, these originate in our early childhood, and are part of our emotional makeup or sense of life.

Statement: "Marriage is so confining that of course I am frustrated."
Response: "What about marriage do you choose to make confining?" "In what way are you frustrated, and what about marriage causes you to choose to be frustrated?"

Statement: "Men are all alike. They just put women down."
Response: "Which man in particular has put you down?" "Have you ever met a man who did not put down a woman?" "In what ways have men exhibited signs of being different from each other, or of being kind to women?"

By examining their perceptions and definitions of their experience of reality, the person has the opportunity to realize that they have created the limitations and they have the power and the ability to redefine what reality could be. This puts the person in control over their response, once again. They will begin to clarify their perceptions, perhaps changing and expanding their definitions of certain axioms.

Deletion

Nominalizations

These are uses of a word that has no intrinsic meaning.

Statement: "He's not being a husband."
Response: "What is a 'husband' to you?"

Statement: "It's hard to change."
Response: "What do you mean by 'hard' and what does 'change' mean to you?"

Unspecified Verbs

The meaning is too ambiguous.

Statement: "She hurt me."
Response: "In what way? Was it emotionally, physically, mentally?"

Statement: "I don't feel well."
Response: "In what way do you not feel well?"

Simple Deletion

The person, thing, or process is missing from the statement. In other words, the referential index is missing.

Statement: "I'm unhappy."
Response: "About what?"

> **Most of the time, neither the fears nor the expectations that people have are based on reality, nor do they ever come to pass.**

Statement: "He's the best."
Response: "Who is? Compared to what or whom?"

Generalization

Universal Quantifiers

These include all, every, never, always, everyone, and no one.

Statement: "They always picked me last."
Response: "Always?" This response addresses the absolute—always. "What would happen if they didn't?" This response elicits new perspectives.

Statement: "I will never give my children sugar."
Response: "Never?" "What would happen if you did?"

Modal Operators of Necessity

These include should, shouldn't, have to, and must.

Statement: "I have to stay in this relationship."
Response: "What would happen if you didn't?"

The person is guided to reconsider their basic beliefs. They look at the axioms, the cause and effect, other possible outcomes, and so forth. Try asking them, "What is the worst thing that would happen if you didn't?" This puts them in the position of facing their greatest fear about the alternatives. Frequently their greatest fear was nebulous and unrealistic.

Modal Operators of Possibility: may, may not, can, cannot, possible, impossible

Statement: "I can't move to another house."
Statement: "What stops you?"

Again, perspectives will be examined to discover that most limitations are self-imposed.

People are powerfully swayed by their constructs based on fear and expectation. These limitations bind them to a narrow path that keeps them running from their fears and pressing towards their positive expectations. When gone unquestioned, we make every choice based on these two things. Learn carefully about these, studying them in yourself and others.

Practice identifying distortions, deletions, and generalizations in your daily conversations. Becoming aware of them will assist you in clarifying your own perceptions of reality, and can be tremendously useful in the healing process for your clients.

Content vs. Process

Content provides the specific details of an event, while process is the basic structure of what happened. In delivering content, you or your client would be naming names, giving the dates, places, emotions involved, quotations from conversations, and so forth. When you or your clients are bogged down in content, learn to discern what is relevant, important, or interesting.

In providing the process, you or your client would describe the outline for steps taken in the event. Should you ever find yourself discussing a case, be sure that you are only revealing the process, not the content of your confidential sessions.

Have you noticed that when people speak in content, their stories are long and the listener frequently begins to tune out? Have you noticed that often the listener is wondering what is the point? With process, the speaker gets to the point rapidly and crisply.

When a client is "hooked" on content, you might wonder why they have the compulsion to include lengthy explanations. Look for clues to justification, rationalization, feeling misunderstood, need for attention, and so forth. Your client may find that by giving long-winded stories with a lot of content, they actually lose the attention of the listener faster, becoming even more frustrated.

In some cases, it will be relevant for you to gently find a way to ask your client, while they are giving their story, "How old do you feel as you tell me this story?" Perhaps you will find that their "inner self" is feeling quite young. This is not necessarily true when the person is a storyteller by trade, nor when the content is relevant and important to conveying the message.

Examples

The following paragraphs are examples to allow you to discern which is content and which is process.

1. "Yesterday Martha and I were at Nordstrom's and decided that we wanted to sit down and have a cup of coffee. We went to Starbucks, and during our conversation, she told me something that really struck a chord. She said, 'My perceptions of reality are shaped by the experiences that I have.'"

2. "Through the many trials of my life I have learned that my experiences shape my perceptions."

3. "When I am working with a client, I would first want them to be comfortable with me and have a sense of trust."

4. "The other day, when my client arrived, I was feeling a little awkward. In fact, I noticed that my hands were sweaty and I had that anxious feeling in my stomach. I didn't want them to know and I especially didn't want them to feel that way, too. I want to be sure that my clients have a sense of trust with me, so I asked my client to sit down so we could talk a little while before we started."

Notice that sentences one and four are laden with content, while two and three are strictly giving process.

Frequently, a question will be much wordier than necessary. Notice the difference between the following two questions, and determine which would be more appealing.

1. "I am interested in learning how to fly airplanes. Can you tell me how much lessons cost?"

2. "When I was a child, my parents took me to Victoria on one of those planes that land on the water. It was so cool and I always thought I would become a pilot. Well, through a series of mishaps, the dream never became a reality until just now. And, because my spouse is working and we're finally doing well enough, I have decided to take up flying. I was wondering how much flying lessons cost."

The flight instructor may have become very impatient with the potential student in example number 2!

Practice discerning when it is important to give content and when process is sufficient and more effective. As a therapist, you will be required to listen to a lot of content from your clients. Often the telling of the story is a big part of the therapy. Over time, you will learn when that is true and when it is unnecessary. When it is not necessary for the healing, or for your edification so that you may help them better, look for signs that they are "stuck" in an earlier age mind frame.

Understanding all the above language patterns will assist your clients in fundamental ways. Practicing these skills in your own life will enhance your proficiency in identifying them and using them in the therapy session.

In later chapters, we will learn how to use these same patterns to induce trance.

CHAPTER 10

Marketing Your Business

All too often, a practitioner receives certification and is surprised that clients are not clamoring at the door for therapy sessions. Marketing a business is a real and important aspect of being self-employed. Make friends with the salesperson within you; perhaps even enhance your confidence to market yourself with the tools you will learn in this book. Whatever you choose to do, please find enjoyable and practical ways of letting people know about your services.

People often feel uncomfortable bragging about themselves. It may be helpful to alter that view of marketing, replacing it with an understanding that you are simply informing people of a service in which they may be interested.

Marketing research shows that a prospective client must be exposed to a brand or product eleven times, on average, before choosing to purchase it. That translates to getting your name and services in front of each individual on eleven occasions before you can expect a response. That seems overwhelming, time consuming, and expensive—and it can be. However, there are smart ways that this can be accomplished with a minimum investment of your time and money.

Try several of the following ideas:

- Write articles for a local newspaper. It is easier to be published in smaller newspapers, targeting ones that have the appropriate audience.
- Teach classes at local venues for continuing education. Try classes in weight loss, smoking cessation, pain management, etc.
- Present workshops. These may be self-generated and marketed or

offered in conjunction with a local shop, bookstore, spa, or healing center.

- Give talks to local civic organizations, sorority houses, and anywhere you can get up in front of a crowd.
- Leave business cards with other complementary health practitioners, such as massage therapists, chiropractors, acupuncturists, aromatherapists, etc. They can then make your cards available to their clients or make referrals.
- Join networking organizations.
- Participate in cooperative ads with other hypnotherapists.
- Give your business card out at every opportunity. Clients can be your hairdresser, favorite waiter/waitress, ski instructor, bartender, etc. People in these professions are also good at sending referrals.
- Participate in health fairs, metaphysical events, trade shows, and such.
- Buy ads in local media—newspapers and radio stations, for instance. These can be costly and may not give as great a return as the aforementioned. However, if professionally designed and wisely placed, they add to your credibility.
- Submit press releases when opening or changing various aspects of your business.

Word of mouth will prove to be your best investment. Give great service, provide positive

> **When they think of hypnotherapy you want them to think of you!**

results in your practice, find a niche that you excel in, and develop and promote the uniqueness that you bring to the field of hypnotherapy.

Money Matters

Setting fees and collecting money for the services provided are touchy subjects for some practitioners. Perhaps they warrant therapy sessions for the therapist!

The fees set for facilitating hypnotherapy should be in line with what the market will bear. They should also be appropriate for the level of expertise and experience being offered. Newly practicing hypnotherapists might consider entering the market at the lower end of the pay scale, while those who have practiced longer, with proven successes, can raise their fees accordingly.

If you provide a service of value, something of equal value must be returned. That may be energy, another service, a product, or money. Without that exchange, several problems will begin to surface.

The providing party may begin to feel used. The receiving party may feel guilty. That alone detracts from the healing

> **Value is an important ingredient in both the healing process and the karmic balance of life.**

being attempted. If the receiving party does not feel guilty, it may only be feeding their syndrome of using other people. Again, this is an unhealthy situation.

If the flow of energy continues in only one direction, eventually the provider will resent the time and energy given and will not want to be available for the receiver. If they do not resent or question the one-way flow of energy, they may only be fostering their own dysfunction of being a martyr or enabler. This is not a very healthy state of affairs for a healer to be in!

When the practitioner is not receiving compensation for their efforts, eventually they will be unable to continue their practice. Then the services will not be available to the clients. In this scenario, everyone loses. As a matter of integrity, all arrangements should be a win-win opportunity.

The issue of money also offers another interesting lesson. Something that is given away has much less value, even in the eyes of the recipient, than something for which they had to invest a considerable amount of money.

When a person is willing to make the call to set up an appointment, agrees to pay the fees, and takes the time and effort to

> **The higher the perceived value of an item or service, the more cherished and useful it is deemed to be.**

show up and participate, you can be assured that they are willing to assist you in making this a productive and successful session. In turn, give them the best that you can offer. Make the session dynamic, be present with your mind and energy as well as your body, and send them out into the world absolutely satisfied that they have spent their money wisely.

PART II

Techniques of Hypnosis

CHAPTER 11

Fundamentals of Hypnotizing a Client

Inductions are the methods by which the hypnotherapist guides clients into a relaxed hypnotic state. There is a wide variety of induction techniques. You are encouraged to become very familiar with the established induction techniques available, and then to experiment with variations, perhaps creating new and interesting methods.

Deepening techniques, which are discussed in a later chapter, are ways to increase the depth of the hypnotic state and to lead, gracefully, into the treatment or therapy most appropriate for the client's presenting problem.

Most induction and deepening techniques could be interchangeable, and can be stacked in any order that facilitates a productive session.

Touching Clients

Many of the induction techniques being taught involve touching the client in some fashion. Although some of these techniques can be highly effective, there are a number of reasons to shy away from touching clients in any way under any circumstances. It is recommended that you consider the following information:

- Having a certification to practice hypnotherapy does not give you a license to have physical contact with your clients. In some states of the U.S., it is explicitly illegal for a hypnotherapist to touch a client unless they have also earned a Massage License or equivalent. Be sure to check your local laws.
- Some clients detest being touched, poked, prodded, hugged, rubbed,

or anything else of that nature. It may be counterproductive to relaxation to touch such a client, invading their personal boundaries and perhaps breaking rapport with them.

• Your touch may be misinterpreted. Remember that you are working with people who are potentially emotionally traumatized, unbalanced, and vulnerable.

• Certain movements can actually injure a client. It may not be obvious that they have a prior weakness or injury that could be exacerbated by movements or touch.

When to Use Inductions

Although highly valuable therapy results have been achieved without the use of formal induction, there will be times when using an induction to lead into other techniques will be advantageous.

Times to use a formal induction include:

• With a first-time client who would expect a formal induction in order to feel they have satisfactorily achieved the hypnotic state

• When a client is particularly distracted, nervous, or tense

• When using suggestion therapy

• When seeking blocked memories

• When the hypnotherapist intuitively senses that it is beneficial

• To achieve the deepest possible states of trance

A formal induction may not be necessary when leading into the session with a somatic or affect bridge, when exploring dreams, when starting the session with Secondary Gains or Parts Therapy, or when the client is already abreacting while you are still in the pretalk phase of the session.

Choosing the Appropriate Induction

Choosing a particular induction technique to use in a given session may be based on one or more of the following:

• The personality of the client—Are they imaginative or analytical? Kinetic or calm? Able to stay focused or easily distracted?

• The environmental conditions—Are there noises in the area or is it quiet and peaceful?

• The client's preference—Have they disclosed that certain inductions

have worked better or worse for them in the past? Have they requested a particular induction?

- The type of therapy to be applied—Will this session be leading to
regression, suggestion, creative visualization, or ego states therapy,
for instance?
- The therapist's preference—Perhaps it is time for a change from previous sessions. By the sixth or seventh client of the day, the hypnotherapist may become bored if repeatedly using the same
induction. It may be time for the hypnotherapist to get out of the routine and stretch their talents in new ways.
- The client's level of resistance to the session—Has the client shown
signs of fear concerning the session or of going into trance? Has rapport been more difficult to establish? Does the client claim to be
unable to "go under"?

The Trance State

The trance state is easily obtained in the normal course of a person's
life. In fact, most people move through their lives in some level of trance.
Frequently the issues of the day—our traumas, crises, trials, and tribulations—are pushed to the side, or are compartmentalized, so that we can
carry on in a way that we would refer to as normal. Thinking we will deal
with them when the time is right, we continue to layer the stresses on top
of one another. The sense of well-being we attempt to create in the midst
of life's issues is just one aspect of the "trance" we experience. This trance
tells us that all is well and safe in the world. This trance convinces us that
we are experiencing life, when in fact we are not being present at all.

**Some trance states that we maintain in our daily lives include
personality traits, self-esteem levels, fears, the need to please others at our own expense, self-sabotaging behaviors, self-sacrifice,
forgetfulness, anger, rage, and even "spacing out."**

Most people who drive cars have experienced missing their exit on the
freeway. Many people have remarked about driving all the way home and
not remembering any part of the trip. That person is said to have been in
trance. Their actions and reactions have been "on automatic."

These are many of the facets of trance. We all do it. We all achieve trance.

When a client claims that they will have difficulty getting into trance, they are simply describing yet another facet of their own trance state. It is their self-description as a person with this trait. It is not necessarily true, and that is easily discovered if they can admit that they have, in fact, been so engrossed in a book or movie that they failed to observe something else happening in the room. Perhaps what they are really communicating to the hypnotherapist is that they resist giving up control, lack trust in the process, have not been comfortable with a particular person attempting hypnosis with them in the past, and so forth.

Using the word trance to describe hypnosis can be essentially misleading. The truth is that the state of hypnosis can actually accomplish a heightened awareness of the here and now. The techniques of hypnosis aim to allow the client to recognize their patterns and beliefs and to eliminate or modify them in an effort to become healthier or happier. However, the term trance is loosely used to describe any altered state of consciousness—whether it is a person's patterns and beliefs or the clarity achieved during a hypnosis session.

The state of hypnosis can be attained with any client. The hypnotherapist may simply have to address the individual's resistance to achieving it. Just as we make time for contemplation and a quiet mind, so too must we set aside time for purposeful hypnotherapy. Such focused presence is not a normal state in our waking hours.

The Client Controls the Depth

Keep in mind that only the client can allow the hypnotic state to occur. Further, only the client can choose to move to deeper levels of trance. If the client resists, you can simply point out that they are exercising control over their lives, proving that there is, in fact, no reason to fear losing control in the session.

When the client affirms that only they can allow themselves to go into trance, and only they can allow the deepest levels of trance to occur, they take responsibility for the success of the session. It is not a matter of the hypnotherapist dragging them from level to level, but their choice to move there willingly.

If there is notable resistance to hypnosis, even when the client has set up an appointment, has shown up, and is willing to pay for it, then the session needs to start right there—addressing the issue of fear and resistance. What is occurring at this point is a type of abreaction. It must be honored and dealt with before the session proceeds in any other fashion. Otherwise, that part of them that is resisting will continue to contaminate any further efforts in the therapy session.

Resistance to the therapy session can easily be handled, to the great relief of both the client and the hypnotherapist. One way is to apply Parts Therapy, which will be discussed in a later chapter.

The Analytical Imp

A successful technique to use with hypervigilant clients is a variation of Parts Therapy. The technique is nicknamed "The Analytical Imp."

At the onset of the hypnosis session, using the techniques for Parts Therapy discussed later in the book, the client is asked to imagine separating the analytical part from the rest of their personality that wants to have an imaginative adventure in hypnosis. When they do that, the analytical part is asked whether it would like to have an even more important job. In commending this part for its purposefulness in the client's life, and complimenting its sense of responsibility and intelligence, we are addressing the ego of that part. When this occurs it is generally most anxious to take on new or different job, especially when it sounds as though it is a promotion!

The following is an example of a script to facilitate this:

"Would you agree that there is a part of you that is analytical and hypervigilant? (Pause for client's concurrence.) *I would like you to imagine separating that part from the rest of you that is interested in having a creative session today. To do this, imagine that the part of you that is analytical is on one of your hands, and the part of you that is imaginative and creative is on the other hand. Tell me when you have done that.* (Pause for client response.)

"I would like to assure that part of you that is analytical that we understand what an important job it has done over the years to assure your safety and survival. We appreciate all that it has accomplished. I am now wondering whether that part of you would be interested in having an even more important job. (Pause for client response.)

"I would like to ask that part of you that is analytical if it would agree to move up to the back of the chair so that it can observe everything that is going on in this session. I wonder if it would be able to pay attention to this session, without being involved in any way. It may find itself becoming curious about what it might feel like to just observe, and pay attention, so that it will have even more information to analyze and think about. Then, at

the end of the session, we can call on it to assist in the process of analyzing what happened. What do you think about that?" (Usually the client says that the part is enthusiastic to have such an important position and that it likes the idea of having more information to process.)

If the part is not yet convinced, continue negotiating. Ask what other concerns it may have, and discover a way to satisfy them.

"I would like to ask the analytical part to now move to the back of the chair as I count from three to one. Three, two, one. How does that feel?"

Proceed with whatever therapy techniques are appropriate to achieve the client's primary goals for the session.

Clients respond well to keeping the Analytical Imp occupied, and frequently request it upon arriving for subsequent sessions. They find relief and relaxation in quieting their mind from its typical busyness.

Creating a Safe Space

Many people find it helpful to create a safe space in which to do their work. This can be envisioned as any place, imagined or real, that allows one to feel relaxed, safe, and free to do what they please.

Frequently, it is beneficial to assist clients in creating their safe space during one of the first few sessions together. This space in a client-centered, nonthreatening atmosphere will be a comforting place for them to retreat to as needed when exploring difficult, emotionally charged, or threatening issues in later sessions.

Script for Creating a Safe Space

"As you close your eyes and take a breath, turn your attention inwards. Search within yourself for that seed of pure spirit that is you. Connect with that part of you that was created at the beginning of time, perfect and radiant. Connect with that part of you now. Feel it; see it.

"Allow that special seed within you to grow brighter as you imagine yourself floating up from your chair. Floating higher and higher. Up through the roof. Floating up through the blue sky, past the clouds. Higher still, past the stars and planets, out into space. That's right. Experience

the vastness of space. Allow your spirit to soar. Imagine your spirit stretching and growing ever more powerful.

"As you begin to float back down towards earth, past the stars, and now past the clouds . . . floating downwards, you see the earth below you. A small blue-green ball, growing ever larger. And as you descend more and more, allow the air moving past you to also move through you. The atoms of the air, flowing through and around all the atoms of your body and soul. Energizing you and carrying away any impurities of thought or intention.

"When a spaceship reenters the earth's atmosphere, the friction creates immense heat and flames. Similarly, as you return to earth, imagine passing through fire. Again, purifying, burning away all that is no longer useful. The fire provides you with energy, passion, and focused intent.

"Continuing your descent, deeper and deeper, you plunge down into a cool and refreshing pond. As the ripples of the water circle concentrically, you sink deep into the water. Relaxed, refreshed. Washing away your cares and negative emotions. Deeper and deeper. Providing comfort and joy, and you float out of the pond and down a gentle river.

"As you float, you begin to notice, along the banks of the river, wondrous scenery, enchanting coves and beaches. Instinctively, you choose a special location, a safe space. Climbing out of the river, and moving into your safe space, you explore and discover many fascinating aspects of this place. And as you examine your location, you find a comfortable place to recline. As you rest comfortably against the earthen floor, you appreciate the soft, yet solid, support offered by the earth. Absorbing the energy of the earth, you feel grounded and secure.

"And now, allowing yourself to go into a deep meditation, you begin to connect with the profound wisdom that is available to you."

At this point, your client can be guided to discover further information concerning their issues and possible healing pathways

There are endless visualizations that can be used to facilitate the creation of a safe space. Be creative and adventuresome!

> **Take a moment to create your own safe space, now. Explore the surroundings and any objects that are included. Notice how you feel as you imagine, create, and enjoy your safe space. Your picture of this place may change over time, or additional spaces may be imagined that serve different purposes.**

CHAPTER 12

Suggestibility Tests

Suggestibility tests allow the client, or a member of an audience, to demonstrate to you—and perhaps more importantly to themselves—their level of ability to be under the spell of their own imagination. During the test, they are responding to an imagined stimulus as though it were happening in the physical world around them.

> **At times, it may be useful, and even entertaining, to present a suggestibility test to your client. Suggestibility tests are also fascinating when you are conducting a group demonstration.**

Suggestibility tests are guided visualizations that elicit overt responses, encouraging people to believe in their own ability to be hypnotized. In a group setting, they allow the hypnotist to discover who will be the best subjects for a demonstration.

Of the many to choose from, here are two that you will find easy and effective. When delivering the suggestions, be as descriptive and dramatic as you can be, so that the client, or audience, is really moved and is in rapport with you.

Tasting Lemons

"As you sit back in your chair, take in a deep breath. As you exhale, allow your eyes to gently close. Allow your attention to turn inwards. Relaxing, releasing, and letting go. And now, I wonder if you can imagine

standing in front of your kitchen counter. Envision yourself there, noticing the colors in your kitchen and the arrangement of your appliances.
Allow yourself to begin to notice the countertop, with a cutting board
placed before you.

"As you continue to observe this scene, you notice a bright yellow,
plump, juicy lemon. It is lying on the cutting board in front of you.

"Imagine taking the lemon in your hands. Feel the texture of its rind
against your fingers. Notice the bright yellow color of its skin. Imagine
the fresh scent of the lemon.

"Laying the lemon on the cutting board, you take a knife and begin to
cut into its skin. You notice the juice squirting out of the fresh, yellow
lemon as you cut through its skin. Soon you have two halves of a fresh
juicy lemon in your hands.

"The aroma of lemon, that fresh bright smell, tantalizes your nostrils
as you bring one of the halves up to your nose and begin to sniff the fresh
juice of the lemon. Something inside of you just can't resist, so you bring
the lemon to your lips and take a nibble of the juicy tart fruit. Once again,
you take a bite of the lemon, remembering the last time that you drank
lemonade or squeezed fresh lemon onto your food. Finding the juice sur-
prisingly tart, you lay the lemon back on the cutting board. The scent of
the lemon oil still fresh on your fingertips. The tart juice is on your lips.

"Having experienced that exhilarating sensation, allow your conscious attention to drift back here to this room, to this time and space.
Now, open your eyes. What did you notice about that experience?"

Most people will be very surprised at how much their mouths salivated. Sometimes it is hard to even lead them through this visualization without frequently having to swallow!

> **Did you notice any response while reading the script?**

Balloons and the Bucket

"Close your eyes and relax. I wonder if you can hold your arms
straight out in front of you, as though you were sleepwalking. As you hold
your arms there, I want you to imagine that I have put a bucket on your
right arm. (Touch the right wrist if that is possible.) Feel the weight of that
bucket as you continue to hold it. (It helps if your voice goes down deep
each time you refer to the bucket.)

"I wonder if you can imagine that I am now tying helium balloons to your left wrist. (Touch the left wrist if possible.) *Feel them as I tie on several great big, colorful helium balloons.* (Allow your voice to rise high in pitch whenever you refer to the balloons.)

"As you focus on the bucket, you notice that I am placing rocks into that bucket. Heavy, heavy rocks. Notice the density and texture of those rocks. Filling the bucket. Getting so heavy.

"And then you notice that there are more and more balloons being tied to your left wrist. Lifting it higher and higher. So light and easy. Notice the colorful shiny surfaces of those helium-filled balloons. Just floating up, up, up with the balloons.

"And the rocks in the bucket are getting so very, very heavy. It is so hard to keep holding the bucket, as it gets heavy . . . so heavy.

"Yet the helium balloons just allow the left arm to float, so easily. Higher and higher, lighter and lighter. Effortlessly, easily, floating up with the balloons.

"And the right arm is so tired. The bucket so heavy. So very difficult to hold the bucket as the rocks grow heavier and heavier. Gravity pulling it downwards. So heavy.

"When you are ready you may open your eyes and see where your arms are now."

You can easily calculate how successful you have been in delivering this visualization. People in the audience will be separating their arms throughout the demonstration. Some people will have arms only slightly separated, while others may have them considerably farther apart. Be wary of those who quickly separate their arms. They may simply be trying to please you, or look successful at the task. When your subjects are truly experiencing it, their arms will slowly separate, haltingly moving in the respective directions.

Suggestibility tests are rarely used in a typical private session. They are useful to know, however, in

> **The greater the response the client has to either of these tests, the more potent access they have to their imagination.**

case someone staunchly denies being able to respond to hypnotic suggestion.

Who Is Suggestible?

It is interesting to note that research in the industry has shown that the people who respond the best to hypnosis and suggestibility tests are those individuals who are intelligent and highly imaginative. This finding is counter to the popular impression that suggestible people have a low level of intelligence or are feebleminded. Children, too, are typically delightful subjects.

Those individuals who are overly analytical or have been diagnosed with attention deficit disorder are more difficult to engage in trance work and suggestibility tests. Even so, many techniques are presented in this book that will easily capture the curiosity and fascination of even the most challenging client. The most difficult clients to work with are the dear souls who are so resistant to the process that they have not made their own appointment for the session. Their spouse or friend has arranged for their therapy.

Always remember that when you exhibit great confidence, it will be shared by your client. Your self-assurance and confidence in the success of the session will provide them with more trust and security about the process.

CHAPTER 13

Techniques of Hypnotic Communication

Earlier in this book, we discovered the covert ways that our clients communicate with us. In this chapter, we will explore strategies for effectively communicating with the conscious and subconscious minds of our clients. Through these techniques, healing and change can occur rapidly and with long-lasting results.

Cause and Effect

There is a natural law of cause and effect. We all live by it and assume its place in our universe. We can, therefore, use it to our advantage during the induction of hypnotic trance. In doing so, we state a cause that is verifiable, followed by an effect that is desired.

Remember that there is great latitude in the creativity and structure of these directives. It is not necessary that they be logical. After all, we are not addressing the rational mind, but rather, the emotional mind.

Cause and effect will utilize the following words:

- Will
- Makes
- Causes
- Forces
- Requires
- Because
- Allows

The following sentences represent a small sampling of the structure of cause and effect clauses.

"The noises you hear around you cause you to go deeper into trance."
"The sound of my voice makes you relax comfortably in your chair."
"Noticing the notes of the music allows your eyelids to grow heavy."
"You arrived in my office safely today because your subconscious mind knows how to take care of you."
"Your well-developed sense of control will allow you to experience an enjoyable state of trance."

Simple Conjunctions

Simple conjunctions link two concepts, creating the sense that they are true by association.

State something verifiable by the client's specific senses, insert a conjunction, and then state the desired behavior. Simple conjunctions use the following words:

- And
- And not
- And do not
- But

Here is a sample of possibilities:

"You are listening to my voice and becoming ever more relaxed."
"People sit in chairs and don't even notice their legs relaxing."
"You are hearing my words but having your own internal visions as well."
"You are breathing and not yet aware of how relaxed you are becoming."

Pacing and Leading

Also referred to as an implied causative, pacing and leading use facts that can be substantiated by the client's sense of reality, then imply a relationship to a desired behavior. It is even more powerful when your sentences are structured so that you verify three or more "facts" in the client's environment and then lead them to the state that you desire to instill.

Pacing and leading will utilize the following words:

- As
- While
- During
- Before

- After
- When
- Following
- Throughout
- Since

Here are examples of pacing and leading:

"As you sit back in the chair, listening to the soft music playing, eyes closed [pacing] . . . you begin to shift into a deeper state of relaxation [leading]."
"While you hear the birds outside the window, and the music playing softly, you continue to breathe naturally [pacing], as your eyelids grow heavy [leading], causing them to gently close [cause and effect] and allowing you to relax even deeper [leading]."
"Since you are here in my office and listening to my voice [pacing], you can easily feel more curious about what you are going to achieve [leading]."

Mind Reading

When accomplished consciously and purposefully, mind reading is a useful tool. These statements will imply that you have insight and knowledge of the internal experiences of the client, whether thoughts or feelings. As you state these "facts," the client must observe their internal experience of the statement, thereby causing the suggestions to become part of the client's actual experience.

For example:

"You must be curious about the emotions that you are experiencing."
"You are becoming aware that you know more than you think you know."
"I know that you are wondering what it will feel like to go into a deeper trance than you have previously experienced."

Notice that the statements are nonspecific and therefore easily attained and verified.

Generalized Referencing

When you use nouns that lack specific referential indices, the client is unable to identify them with themselves or their own situation. Therefore, their subconscious mind may learn from the story or metaphor without the filtering or protective blocks that would more likely occur if the words were directed to them.

In this category, the following words will be used:

- People
- Someone
- They
- One
- A friend
- A client
- Something
- Everyone

"A client once told me that nothing was wrong, when she was actually feeling quite sad."
"Someone once said, 'The burden is lighter when shared by two people.'"
"Trees know how to bear fruit in their own time."
"Some people emerge from trance feeling wonderfully relaxed and refreshed."

Deletion

When the specific nouns and the referential indices are removed, the meaning of the phrase becomes obscure and incomplete. This allows clients to fill in the details with their own meaning, making sense of the message in a way that is specific to them.

". . . and you may find it satisfying . . ."
". . . moving through the experience . . ."
". . . sensing this change in ways that allow you . . ."

Nominalizations

Again, these nonspecific words sound substantial, yet allow for a range of definitions specifically relevant to the client.

Words in this category include:

- Sense, sensation

- Aware, awareness
- Relax, relaxation
- Comfort, comfortable
- Satisfy, satisfaction
- Know, knowledge
- Experience
- Express
- Notice

Sample visualizations using nominalizations are:

"As you move through this space, you begin to notice the sensations that come into your experience."
"As you notice the sounds around you, you allow yourself to become aware of your knowledge and wisdom."

Nothing specific has actually been said, yet the client will create a sensory-rich experience that is uniquely of their own creation.

Ambiguity

This technique involves the use of the English language in such a way that several meanings can be attached to the word or phrase.

1. Phonological Ambiguity—The use of different words that sound the same:

- Apart—a part
- Wait—weight
- Knows—nose
- There—their—they're
- Are—our—hour
- You—hue
- Read—red
- Here—hear
- A parent—apparent
- Light—As in color, weight, or luminescence
- A jar—ajar
- Know—no

For example:

"I wonder when you will notice you are light." "I wonder when you will notice your light."
"When you open your eyes, notice the new hue." "When you open your eyes, notice the new you."

2. Syntactical Ambiguity—When the context of the word is open to interpretation.

- "I hope the weight/wait is not a problem to you."
- "When they become apparent/a parent to you."

3. Ambiguity of Scope—When it cannot be determined whether a word relates to a part or the entire sentence.

- "Our honored guests and members."
- "Old men and women."
- "Can you draw a picture of yourself in a Halloween costume?"

4. Ambiguity through Punctuation—When the punctuation is removed between two well-formed sentences that share a common word or words.

- "Notice where you placed your hand me that paper."
- "There is beauty in all that you look at how far you have come."

Playing with words, and using them to great advantage within the hypnosis session, can be creative and entertaining. Although it seems like a lot of information to remember, study the categories one at a time, tackling a new one as each is mastered. Before long, the language patterns will be second nature.

CHAPTER 14

Induction Techniques

Many techniques and styles can be used for the induction of hypnotic trance. Choosing the most suitable one for a given session is dependant on taste, application, and the effect you wish to create.

As you learn and practice the techniques, they will naturally become stylized. That is perfectly acceptable. The techniques are not as important as the results they are meant to produce. Learn them, play with them, and find ways to customize them to suit your client's needs!

Progressive Relaxation

The Progressive Relaxation induction is an industry standard. It can be very effective and most clients find it particularly relaxing. One positive aspect of the Progressive Relaxation induction is that it gives focus to the body. People are frequently disconnected from their bodies to some degree. It is possible that they have not paid a great deal of attention to it in quite some time. It is common for people to simply ignore little aches, pains, tension, and stress. When the client's attention is drawn, slowly, from part to part along their body, they have the opportunity to really honor that part and to specifically concentrate on giving it some needed relief and relaxation.

How often do we dismiss our backside, or ignore our extremities? Most of us are simply unaware of the tightness in the fine, deep muscles around our eyes and foreheads that we keep squinted and furled throughout the day. This induction procedure allows for a thorough release of even the forgotten parts of our physical selves.

> **Progressive relaxation is appropriate most anytime; however, it can be particularly helpful in cases of anxiety, pain, panic, and stress.**

Progressive Relaxation is easy, because, as a hypnotherapist, you simply have to start at the head or the toes, and name the successive body parts. Remember to speak slowly, soothingly, and rhythmically. The tone and tempo of your voice add subtle coaxing to the relaxation process. If you speak in a rapid, loud, or choppy manner, it will be counterproductive to creating a calm and peaceful state in your client.

As stated above, you can begin at the head or the feet. Feel free to alternate them. The benefit of starting at the toes, and coming upwards, is the energies are more focused in the head at the end. After all, it is the head—including the mind, brain, and intuition—that we are going to be working with. When starting at the head and going downwards, consider using a deepening technique, such as the Ball of Light, that brings the focus back up to the forehead (see the next chapter).

Sample Script for the Progressive Relaxation Induction

"Sit back . . . and when you are ready, you can simply allow your eyes to close. Taking a nice, deep breath. (Breathe in with them.) *Ahhh, yes, just releasing any tension as you exhale.*

"Continuing to relax deeper and deeper with every breath, feeling the air moving in and refreshing . . . and moving out, relaxing. That's right. Just letting go.

"And now, relaxing your toes and your feet . . . your ankles and your calves. Relaxing and letting go.

"Relaxing your knees and your thighs, allowing your legs to just release and relax. Just letting go. That's right.

"And I know that you are already aware that you are the only one who can truly allow you to relax, to release your muscles. You are the only one who can truly allow yourself to go as deeply into relaxation as you possibly can. And you can go there now.

"Relaxing your stomach, your chest, and your breathing. And perhaps you notice the rhythm of your breathing as it finds its own natural pace. (Be silent for about three breaths.)

"Relaxing your shoulders, your arms, your hands, and your fingers. That's right, just letting go. Feeling so good to be doing something so good just for you. Just relaxing, releasing, and letting go.

"You know that only you can give yourself permission to relax more thoroughly than you have ever relaxed before. That's right. Enjoying it. Knowing that the rest of the world will simply continue to function normally for this next hour as you allow yourself to do something that is just for you.

"Feeling so good. So curious."

From here, move to the deepening technique of the Ball of Light. Or continue:

"I wonder if you can relax your neck. Just letting it support your head, yet relaxing any unnecessary tension. Just letting go. Relaxing so deeply. That's right. Very good.

"And now, relaxing all the muscles in your face. That's right. All the muscles around your jaw and ears. Relax the muscles around your mouth, your nose. All the fine muscles around your eyes. That's right, those fine muscles deep inside. Just relaxing. And now, releasing your forehead. That's right, all the fine muscles are just letting go, relaxing and releasing. That's right."

At this point, you may choose to administer a deepening technique, to achieve an even greater depth of relaxation. You may also use creative visualization to facilitate the passage from your direct suggestions (of relaxation) to their active participation in therapy.

Dave Elman Induction

This powerful induction takes the client into a deep state of hypnotic trance. This is the induction of choice when the plan is to use suggestion therapy or any other technique that requires a deep level of trance. This works well for those clients who are hypervigilant and highly analytical, and requires the client to take responsibility for their levels of relaxation and trance.

It is important when using the Dave Elman induction to achieve success at each step before proceeding to the next one.

Before beginning, it is advisable to ask the client for permission to touch their wrist during the induction. If the client is not comfortable with that, the hypnotherapist must revise the induction accordingly. It is more often the case that the client will give permission.

The following is a stylized version of the Dave Elman induction:

"As you sit back in the chair, just take in a long, deep breath. Hold it . . . and now as you exhale, allow your eyes to close. (Client's eyes close.) And now you can simply focus on all the muscles around your eyes. All the fine little muscles. Just allowing them to relax, releasing them, so deeply. That's right. Just relaxing. Feeling the eyelids so relaxed that as long as you maintain this level of relaxation, your eyelids simply will not open. Even if you were to attempt to open your eyes. That's right. So relaxed.

"And, when you realize that you have relaxed your eyelids deeply, you can test them. Simply maintaining this deep relaxation . . . trying to open your eyes . . . that's right . . . test them."

> **All responses are correct.**

If the client opens their eyes, assure them of their success by saying, *"Very good. You have shown yourself that you are able to control what happens to you. That's good. And now you can also allow yourself to achieve even greater satisfaction, knowing that you can allow yourself to truly relax them so completely that as long as you don't remove that relaxation, they simply won't open at all. Now let's try again. Closing your eyes. Relaxing."* (If the client tries to open their eyes and they remain closed, assure them that they have done very well. Then continue.)

"Now that you have achieved this wonderful sensation of relaxation in your eyelids, I wonder if you can bring that sense of relaxation up to the top of your head, and then just allow it to flow down over you. Over your entire body, like a wave of relaxation, flowing, relaxing, releasing. That's right. Very good.

"Now this sense of relaxation can deepen even further. In a moment, I am going to ask you to open and close your eyes. When you do so, that is your signal to really let go, deepening this sense of relaxation ten times greater. All you have to do is to want it to happen, and to let it happen. Now go ahead and open . . . and close . . . your eyes. That's right.

"Feel the relaxation flowing throughout your body, taking you deeper and deeper. All the way down. Use your imagination and enjoy this wonderful sensation. Very good.

"We can deepen this relaxation even more. Again, I am going to ask you to open and close your eyes. Again as you do so, allowing yourself to double your relaxation again. Now open and close your eyes. Going all the way down. Deeper and deeper. Allowing every muscle in your body to relax so deeply that as long as you maintain this relaxation, your muscles simply will not work.

"Once more, when I ask you to open and close your eyes, you will do so, allowing your relaxation to double once again. Going so deep . . . feeling so good. Now, go ahead and open . . . and close . . . your eyes. That's right. Going all the way down. Deeper and deeper.

"In a moment, I am going to test how very relaxed your body truly is, by simply raising your right [or left] arm. (Take a hold of the client's wrist.)

"I want you to remain as relaxed as you are right now . . . and allow me to do all the work, as I lift your arm. (Lift the arm.) *Letting me support all the weight. That's right. No need to assist me in any way. Just relaxing. Letting me do the work.* (Gently move the arm to see if it hangs from your support in a relaxed and natural manner.)

"In a moment, I'm going to drop your arm into your lap. I would like you to simply allow it to drop naturally, maintaining this wonderful state of relaxation. OK, dropping your arm. Very good. So relaxed. (Observe whether the arm drops limply, or if they seem to guide it down.)

"Now, I'm going to check that arm one more time, to really allow you to relax even deeper. Really letting go . . . that's right . . . very good. Letting me have all the weight this time. Really heavy. (Lift and drop the arm once more, again watching for any control they are exerting.)

"Now that you have shown yourself that you can relax your body so deeply, I'd like to see if you can also allow your mind to become just as relaxed. Yes, relaxing your mind, and your thoughts.

"So, I would like you to follow my instructions. In a moment, I will ask you to count backwards from 100. With each number that you say I want you to repeat, 'Deeper relaxed.' And with each number, simply pushing the remaining numbers out of your head. Just forgetting the numbers, relaxing them away. So that before you get to the number 97 . . . or maybe even sooner . . . the numbers will have simply faded away, pushing them right out of your head. So it will be like this . . . 100 . . . deeper relaxed . . . 99 . . . deeper relaxed. Pushing the numbers out, they will simply disappear . . . fade . . . your mind relaxing them away. Now you can do it."

Allow the client to begin the exercise of counting. You can encourage their ability to forget the numbers, reminding them to simply push them out of their heads, as they go deeper and deeper.

When they are finished, you may continue with a deepening technique or begin suggestion therapy, ideomotor and ideosensory techniques, or another therapy technique of your choice.

This induction consistently produces very successful results. It can even be used in the middle of a session if the client needs to be taken deeper for a special exercise, or if they have begun to emerge prematurely and you want them to go back into trance even deeper.

Ericksonian Confusion Technique

This interesting technique has produced mixed reviews among clients and students. Some love it, while others find it agitating. When using this technique in a session, you may wish to explain it in advance so the client does not spend the time wondering if they are failing because they are lost. Being lost is part of the desired result.

This technique is generally most enjoyed by imaginative, light-hearted people. It is most despised

> **It may be helpful to record this onto a cassette tape and experience it firsthand.**

by analytical people who are vigilant and fearful of losing control. Both groups can greatly benefit from the technique, which is aimed at occupying the analytical hemisphere of the brain while activating the creative hemisphere.

The methodology is that the phrases sound as though they make sense. The analytical part of the person is grasping for meaning and logic. However, the strings of phrases are not logically meaningful. Over time, the analytical part of the brain tires of the attempt and has to "check out," leaving the imagination to run wild.

This is particularly effective when implanting productive suggestions, as the brain finds comfort in grasping onto any verbalization that seems to be logically constructed. It is much like grabbing onto a buoy of safety in a sea of chaos. If there are useful suggestions to create for the client, they can be done about three-quarters of the way through the script sequence. When clients or students experiencing this technique emerge from this state, they remark that they were aware that a suggestion was being made and that it felt good and right at the time, and yet they cannot remember what the suggestion was.

The induction is constructed here as a graph so that the hypnotherapist has the liberty to mix and match words and phrases from whichever column, randomly and with wild abandonment of making any real sense to the logical mind.

If you choose to tape-record a bit of this, try speaking at a normal, or slightly slower, speed, and then again at an excruciatingly slow speed. Notice the difference in your experience as you listen to the tape. One of the most difficult parts in delivering this induction is allowing enough silence between the words and phrases to emphasize the level of confusion.

Client Experience

Some clients will be concerned that they failed in the process because their minds wandered—almost dreamlike—to bizarre and disjointed thoughts and fantasies. That phenomenon is a natural, and desirable, side effect of this technique. There is a lot to sort through and discover that has been stored in the subconscious mind—and this confusion technique can aid in the discovery of some of that material. It may be likened to inducing wakeful dreaming.

On that same note, it may be dangerous to use this technique with someone who has been medically diagnosed as, or is suspected of being, psychotic, or has suffered posttraumatic stress disorder or multiple-personality disorders, or is in any other way susceptible to the negative effects of disorientation.

Using the Monologue Graph

The table on page 104 provides a selection of phrasing for the Confusion Monologue. Keep it handy to refer to while delivering the induction. Over time, you will find other words to add to this collection. Read the lines straight across, or deviate from the norm, circling around the columns in a free-flowing manner. Continue for about five to twenty-five minutes, watching for physical signs of the client's level of relaxation and altered state of consciousness. Five minutes would be sufficient when leading into a deepening technique, or using it as such. Continuing for twenty-five minutes or longer is beneficial when the session consists primarily of silent self-discovery, implanting suggestions, inducing sleep for insomniacs, and allowing the person time for creative mental play.

Ericksonian Environmental Induction

This wonderful induction technique is easily administered anywhere, anytime. There is no script to read or memorize. It is simply an observation of the environment and the client's verifiable experience.

The key to this induction is that the phrasing you choose must be real and verifiable to the client. Should it deviate from your client's sense of reality, you will break rapport with them and hinder the induction process.

The benefits of this induction, other than being readily available, are:

• A heightened sense of observation
• Increased rapport when applied properly
• Directing the focus of the client's attention without being authoritarian or threatening
• Allows noises and other distractions in the environment to become part of, instead of a deterrent to, the session

The general guidelines for applying this induction technique are:

• Start with obvious experiences the client senses, beginning farther away from the client and moving closer.
• Stay aligned with verifiable experience.
• Incorporate as many senses as possible: temperature, smells, sounds, etc.
• Partway through, begin to incorporate curiosity, wonderment, and possibilities.
• Towards the end, initiate gentle leading by using simple conjunctions, implied causative, and cause and effect statements, which were previously discussed.

This technique can be used in any session. A shortened version may lead to another induction or deepening, or a longer version may lead right into a therapy technique.

Sample of the Environmental Technique

"Closing your eyes and relaxing against the chair, perhaps you begin to become aware of the birds outside the window, singing. And the notes of the music coming from the stereo. As you allow your mind to float on those notes, just drifting and relaxing, you may also be aware of the voices

Confusion Monologue

Imagine if you were to	notice	the depth
Can you	touch	the difference
Perhaps you can	access	the comfort
You might	enjoy	the logic
When will you	comprehend	the imagery
I wonder if you can	understand	the significance
Will you be able to	remember	the change
Might you	sense	the connection
Would you	see	the purpose
Do you notice how you can	listen to	the metaphor
You may or may not	trust	the possibility
You might enjoy the	observe	the vastness
It's nice to	satisfy	the respect
One could	imagine	representations
Where do you	hear	the expanse
You know how to	taste	the delight
You may wish to	desire	the uniqueness
No need to	relax into	the meaning
How will you know when you	find	the reality
What happens when you	enter	the passion
Will you be able to	believe in	the answers
It may be confusing to	hide	the intention

within	curiosity	and	experience
surrounding	wisdom	whenever	integrity
revealed by	balance	through	certainty
encompassing	dreams	during	choice
traversing	contemplation	except by	passion
fulfilled by	logic	where there is	connection
found in	purpose	throughout	guidance
that accommodates	creativity	along with	truth
that co-creates	resourcefulness	because of	evolution
running through	space	or	ambiguity
flowing through	confidence	also	reality
secured by	time	as well as	trance
of	paradox	while	transformation
behind	growth	but	freedom
hidden by	exploration	if	independence
revealed by	humor	as with	love
inherent in the	unconsciousness	even through	peace
embraced by	commitment	meanwhile	spirituality
leading to	completion	enhancing	knowledge
between	harmony	as if	solutions
during	awareness	behind	imagery
contained in	silence	around	consciousness

coming from the hallway. These voices simply serve to remind you to go deeper inside, relaxing and releasing. And perhaps you notice the sound of footsteps overhead, knowing that it is a natural part of the office environment. Relaxing. Knowing that the world continues to function just the way it should, even while you are relaxing and taking care of you.

"A part of you has noticed the sound of the air coming through the vents, and the temperature of the air against your face and hands. Being so aware and yet so relaxed, and comfortable. Feeling so good. That's right.

"As you notice the way that your shirt feels as it rests against your skin, and the way that the soles of your feet feel as they rest against the floor, you know that it feels good to relax all the way down. Deeper and deeper.

"And I wonder if you have become curious about what this experience will be like for you. And perhaps you wonder how very deeply you will allow yourself to go. Just relaxing and releasing. Knowing that only you can really allow yourself to go deeper than you have ever gone before. Relaxing. Feeling so calm and safe . . . so comfortable. Have you ever noticed the difference in sensation between your right hand and your left? Or contemplated the distance between your right ear and your left? And as you focus on that now, relaxing, in wonderment, I wonder if you have noticed the possibilities that lie before you, the choices."

From here, simply continue with more experiences, or move into a deepening technique or directly into therapy.

The Ericksonian Environmental induction technique is highly portable. It is available to be used anywhere and in any situation. When you include the events and situations surrounding the client, instead of attempting to block them out artificially, a noise is not considered a distraction, but rather is enveloped into the experience in a smooth and comforting way.

Discover More

There are many, many more induction techniques. Some are established, and some are yet to be discovered. Over time, you will encounter new methods of inducing hypnosis, and you may even create some very effective methods of your own. Avoid letting your sessions become dull or stale. Keep adding new and different techniques to fascinate your client, expand your skills, and make the sessions interesting for you.

CHAPTER 15

Techniques for
Deepening the Trance

Deepening the trance creates greater relaxation for the client and allows them to achieve a fuller connection with the subconscious mind.

Deepening the trance is particularly important when the hypnotherapist is planning to use suggestion therapy. It also helps achieve greater success in exercises that involve memory, imagination, and the discovery of information and patterns. Deepening techniques are useful too when you are working with clients who get in their own way, through overanalyzing, critical thinking, and self-doubts.

Again, deepening techniques and inductions are frequently interchanged. Deepening techniques generally involve guided imagery, visualization, and any style of language that directs the client from a relaxed state to a lower level of brainwave cycles. Yet it may be considered a higher level of awareness. The client's attention can either become much more focused and exclusive or much broader and inclusive.

When to Apply Deepening Techniques

Use deepening techniques when:

- The client has difficulty relaxing
- The client is easily distracted
- The client needs assistance in the creative visualization process
- The hypnotherapist chooses to use suggestion therapy
- The session involves memory recall or elevated somatic or affective content

- The client shows signs of not having reached an appropriate level of relaxation to begin therapy techniques

The Hallway

The Hallway deepening technique is a classic for several reasons:

- It accesses client-created visual and kinesthetic material, which starts the process of tuning into their senses more fully.
- It allows the client to create a scene, through their imagination, that has no right or wrong answers.
- It is nonthreatening.
- The doors allow the client to have choices.

Sample Script for the Hallway Deepening

"I wonder if you can imagine a hallway, stretching out in front of you. This hallway can look like anything you choose. It may be a hallway that you have seen at one time, and it may be a hallway that you have created completely out of your imagination."

Most people have no problem making up a hallway. However, when you give them the choice to make it up or remember one, those who consider themselves to have poor imaginations will have the alternative to visualize one they have seen, and avoid what they may consider a failure.

"And as you begin to move down along this hallway, you begin to notice the texture of the floor covering beneath your feet, and the color of the walls."

Be sure to keep your language nonleading. Use "move" rather than "walk," as some clients may see themselves floating or crawling. Use "the texture" rather than "the roughness or smoothness," which may disagree with the vision that they are having. Use the term "color" rather than "light/dark/red/beige," etc., once again avoiding a disagreement with the client's experience.

"And there are doorways along this hall, each one leading to information . . . and experiences . . . that will be so helpful in understanding the issues that we have been discussing today."

Avoid telling them the number of doorways that they will notice unless there is a specific reason why there would only be a certain number, such as when exploring the possible futures of two divergent life paths. Even then, if the client sees three doors, there may be a choice that neither of you had considered as a possibility, and one that certainly will be worth exploring.

"And as I count from three to one, you will find yourself in front of one of those doors . . . three . . . two . . . one.
"Remaining this relaxed and yet able to speak, how would you describe the door that you find yourself in front of?"

Advising them that they are able to speak cues them that it is their turn to verbalize their experience. Clients who have not had experience with this type of therapy sometimes don't understand that they are expected to respond aloud.

Wait for the client's response. Allow them to fully describe the door. This encourages the client's transition from listening to your directives to accessing and creating their own experience.

"What else do you notice about this door?
"Do you notice anything else?"

Sometimes the description of the door gives clues as to the content to be discovered beyond it. Are they describing it as old, modern, with a window, or as a tightly locked steel door?

"Are you ready to open this door and step through?"

Always ask if they are ready. This keeps the session client centered. They may be anxious to explore, or they may hesitate or even fear what they will find upon opening the door. If the client expresses either hesitation or fear, don't push them to proceed. Take time to explore their feelings and what they expect to find beyond the door. Remember that there is a part of them that already knows what is beyond that door. Sometimes their fears are well founded—they will be exploring a highly sensitive event— and sometimes the fears are exaggerated beyond what could really happen should they cross that threshold. It is imperative that the fears are explored and the client is feeling safe and prepared to proceed.

It is not unheard of for the entire remainder of the session to be spent dealing with the fear of proceeding. If it goes that way, so be it. The client's sense of security and trust, in both you and in the process, will dictate the success of your future relationship and work together.

When the client says they are ready:

"Go ahead and open the door and step through. What do you begin to notice around you?"

Again, some clients will begin a descriptive commentary about their visions, feelings, or experiences, while other clients will claim they don't see anything. Stay client centered. Even blackness may have metaphorical significance. Work with them to discover the quality of the darkness, or how they feel about being in that particular darkness, and so forth.

From this point, the hypnotherapist can proceed with the therapy technique of their choice.

The Elevator Deepening Technique

> **Before using this technique, determine whether your client has a phobia about elevators. If so, this visualization will be highly unproductive in furthering or deepening trance!**

"Imagine yourself in front of an elevator door. It can look like anything you choose. It may be an elevator that you have seen before, or it may be one that you have created in your imagination.

"As you continue to observe this elevator, you notice the elevator door opening.

"As you allow yourself to step onto the elevator, you find it comfortable and relaxing.

"Out of curiosity, you look at the control panel. You notice that you are on the top floor—the fifth floor. And as the door closes, you notice that the elevator begins to descend, going down . . . down . . . down. As the elevator continues to move downwards, you find it so comforting to relax even deeper . . . going down . . . going deeper.

"And as the elevator comes to a stop at the fourth floor, the door opens. You find it relaxing to simply remain on the elevator. You notice the scene that lies beyond the door, passively observing, remaining on the elevator.

*As the door closes, the elevator begins to move downwards again . . .
deeper and deeper . . . going down . . . so relaxing.*

*"The elevator comes to rest at the third floor. The door opens, and you
find it so easy—simply observing the scene that lies beyond the door.
Remaining on the elevator as the door once again closes. Again, you
begin to notice the movement of the elevator . . . going down . . . deeper
and deeper . . . so relaxed . . . so comfortable.*

*"And the elevator arrives at the second floor. The door opens. Once
again you observe the scene that is occurring beyond the door, remaining
on the elevator, as the door begins to close. The elevator moving . . . deeper and deeper . . . so relaxing . . . so fascinating . . . as it moves now . . .
to the deepest level . . . all the way down now.*

*"As you notice the elevator arriving at the first floor . . . so deep . . .
so comforting . . . and the elevator door opens, this time . . . you exit the
elevator. As you do so, what do you begin to experience?"*

The Elevator is an interesting deepening technique, which can easily be
used as an induction all on its own. My clients have not only enjoyed this,
on occasion they have guided the session back to other scenes that they
viewed at the different levels or "floors," each scene contributing relevant
information to the issue being explored.

The Stairway Deepening Technique

The Stairway is an obvious and well-used technique for deepening. It
may be set up in many ways. The hypnotherapist may determine the sensory details and/or the exact number of stairs or may leave these open to
the client's imagination. It is preferable to be nonleading in the description of the stairs, yet to determine the number of steps, to keep track of
where the client is in the process.

Further, the hypnotherapist may wish to establish where the client
lands at the bottom of the stairs, or they may also want to leave that up to
the imagination of the client. Always stay as nonleading as possible and
encourage the imaginative participation of the client.

A Sample Stairway Deepening

*"As you continue to relax in your chair, I wonder if you can imagine a
stairway leading downwards. That stairway can look like anything that*

you wish. It may be a stairway that you are familiar with, or it may be one created from your imagination.

"As you approach the top of that stairway, you look downwards, noticing that there are ten steps to the bottom . . . to the deepest levels. Relaxing, and feeling so curious. And as you continue to observe these stairs, you know, you can sense, that with each step downwards, you, too, will relax deeper and deeper. Each step going down . . . more relaxed . . . deeper in trance.

"So, as you step onto that tenth step . . . downwards . . . going deeper . . . you may find it interesting how easy it is to allow yourself to go deeper into relaxation. Deeper . . . more comfortable . . . that's right.

"Going to the next step, nine . . . going even deeper. Doubling your relaxation. That's right . . . just letting go.

"And taking the eighth step, you may discover yourself going even deeper . . . and deeper. So relaxed . . . and feeling so good.

"And on the seventh step . . . just letting go. That's right . . . deeper and deeper.

"Sixth step. Doubling your relaxation once again. Finding it so curious just how deeply relaxed you can allow yourself to go.

"Fifth step. That's right. Relaxing even deeper. Very good. Just allowing it to happen.

"Fourth step. Going deeper and deeper. Knowing only you can allow yourself to relax so well.

"Third step. Letting it happen. And I wonder if you will go deeper in trance than you have ever experienced. That's right . . . very good. . . .

"Second step. Almost there. Doubling your trance once again. Going all the way down now.

"First step. So relaxed. All the way down. That's right. And as you find yourself at the final level, you begin to realize that when you take the final step, you will be on the bottom floor. All the way down. Arriving there now.

"And as you take that step to the lowest level . . . relaxing into it . . . you discover where you are. And as you explore your surroundings with the curiosity of a child, you begin to learn about this environment. And remaining this relaxed, and yet able to speak, what do you notice about where you are now?"

Allow the client to describe to you where they are. Once again, if the final step put them into a space that is all dark or all light, inquire as to their experiences about that darkness or lightness. Is it a closed or open feeling? Are they comfortable or not? What emotions do they experience while finding themselves here? These questions can then allow the hypnotherapist to lead into a somatic or affect bridge to another time they had a similar feeling. Alternatively, the hypnotherapist may choose to have them make up a story about this darkness, leading them into a Reverse Metaphor.

The Stairway deepening technique is conducive to regression and the discovery of blocked memories, among other goals.

Ball of Light Deepening Technique

This is an enjoyable technique, easy to use, that continues the relaxation process as it draws the client's energies and focus upwards to the head. The Ball of Light technique ignites the imagination and the visualization processes. It energizes the forehead, helping connect the conscious and subconscious minds and stimulating each.

The graceful application of the Ball of Light deepening is enhanced in combination with two others, in this order: Progressive Relaxation, Ball of Light, and then the Hallway deepening, leading into the dialogue segment of the therapy session. This is a smooth and generally successful means of encouraging the client's use of imagination and visualization.

Sample Script for the Ball of Light Deepening

"I wonder if you can imagine a ball of light at your feet, glistening, shining, and radiating.

"And as that ball of light begins to move up along your body, it begins to gather up the perceptions and sensations, leaving behind a completely relaxed body.

"As it moves up along your legs and across your lap, and now across your torso, your energies and focus move upwards. That's right.

"Allow that ball of light to move up, now across your throat, clearing and balancing your energies. Moving on up, right on up, to the center of your forehead. That's right. Very good.

"And as the ball of light begins to energize this area of the forehead, you may begin to notice the sensation as it begins to open and expand, the energy flowing through, connecting the conscious mind to the subconscious mind. That area of your mind that houses the knowledge that will be so pertinent to the issues that we were discussing just moments ago.

"I will now invite the subconscious mind to begin to prepare that information that will be so interesting and useful in the discovery of the issues, their origins, and the means to resolve them."

From here, the client can be directed into the hallway, as you say, *"I wonder if you can imagine a hallway."* Or you can count, by saying, *"As I count from ten to one, your subconscious mind will begin to share with your conscious mind that information."* Alternatively, you may choose to lead directly into a hypnotherapy technique of your choice.

The Ball of Light deepening technique has even worked well on its own with repeat clients who are known to go into their visualizations rather easily. It can also be used as a quick relaxing and focusing tool when the hypnotherapist is planning to use a therapy tool that would not necessarily need a lengthy or formal induction.

This technique can be applied to oneself when preparing for meditation, or at bedtime when desiring to program oneself to remember one's dreams. Clients can easily be taught this technique for use in self-hypnosis, increasing visualization skills, decreasing insomnia, and more.

Discover and Create
the Best Method for Your Session

As can be seen, there are many ways for a person to enter the trance state. The method chosen will be left to the discretion of the hypnotherapist or the preference of the client. Feel free to experiment with the various techniques and styles, discovering for yourself which ones you are comfortable with and which ones give you the desired results.

This is by no means a complete list of inductions and deepening methods. Over time, you may discover new ones that you will want to try or ideas that will allow you to develop your own style and technique.

CHAPTER 16

Completing the Hypnosis Session

At the end of a hypnosis session, there are many ways to bring the client back to wakefulness. Most styles consist of instructing the client that they will return to alert awareness by whatever words or signals the therapist is going to administer. That may include snapping the fingers, counting from one to five, or uttering a specific word.

To reiterate an earlier statement, there is no danger that the client will be unable to emerge from hypnosis. If they are so deep that they don't respond, which is quite rare, they will simply awaken at the end of a short sleep cycle.

Preferred Strategy for Emerging from Trance

- Inform the client that the session is about to end
- Ask the client if there is anything else they feel is necessary to be completed before finishing the session
- Explain that as you count from one to five they will return to normal wakefulness
- Give appropriate posthypnotic suggestions
- Begin the process of counting
- Sit quietly with the client as they readjust to awareness of the office space
- Conclude with a discussion of how they feel, asking if there are any questions or concerns to address

Sample Script for Emergence from Hypnosis

"We are nearing the end of our session. Is there anything else that needs to be addressed or completed before we finish for today?

(Typically, the client will say no; however, if they do say yes, take a few moments to satisfy that request.)

"In a moment I will count from one to five, bringing you back to this present time and space. Before we do that, I would like to remind you that you will remember all that we have done and said in this session. Asking the subconscious mind to continue the work that we have begun today, continuing to reveal to your conscious mind even more wisdom and deeper understanding of these issues in the days and weeks to come. Continuing to manifest the changes and healing initiated in this session. And now, returning here, as I count . . . one . . . two . . . three . . . coming up . . . four . . . aware of this time and space . . . and five, fully alert . . . and enthusiastic about the path that lies before you."

In this emergence script, the hypnotherapist has remained very client centered. The client has been alerted to what is coming next, and the needs of the client have been addressed by asking if there is anything more to do. Instructions have been given to the subconscious and conscious minds as to their expected roles, both now and in the near future. Then the counting begins, with gentle direction to return to the normal state of awareness.

> **Notice the use of the word "aware" rather than "awake." This supports the notion that hypnosis is an altered state, rather than a sleep state.**

As you begin to count, allow your voice to move from the flowing, soft, hypnotic-trance voice to brighter, more lilting, energized, conversational tones. This gives the client an additional signal of the direction in which they are going.

Posthypnosis Discussion

While your client is emerging from hypnosis, be respectful of their mental state, continuing to retain rapport.

Sit quietly and allow them to signal when they are ready to have a discussion. When they are ready, ask them if they have any questions or comments about their experience. Be sure to answer their questions and give them instructions on how they may integrate what they have learned into their daily routines. Many people are confident they know

> **Assure your clients that should any questions arise after they leave your office, they are welcome to call or e-mail.**

how to proceed, while some clients need assistance in putting their experiences into context and practical application.

Concerns, confusion, or further emotional abreaction may be delayed until clients are in their normal environments. It is helpful for them to know that they can obtain answers and support long after their appointment.

Notes for Future Sessions

While the client is emerging from trance, or shortly after they leave your office, take the opportunity to make additional notes in the file with suggestions for topics that would be appropriate in subsequent sessions. These may include subjects that were brought up in session but not addressed, or those that were not completed during the session. Your notes may also include ideas of therapy techniques you think will be helpful in future sessions. If you are giving a referral to a specialist, such as a psychologist, naturopath, or body worker, make a note of that as well. Any books or agencies you suggest should also be listed.

Remember that time will pass and your focus will be on many other clients before you see this person again. Do not rely on your memory for the details of each case.

Future Appointments

At the close of the session, you may also discuss with your client the need or desire for future appointments. If possible, set the next appointment at that time. When they get back to work and home, they may become so immersed in other activities that they will forget to take care of themselves until another crisis occurs. Explain to them that they will be supporting their investment in themselves and their health by continuing the healing process through to completion.

When you are seeing clients with addiction disorders, it is crucial to maintain the supportive therapies until the change is complete. Some clients want to experience the positive results gained from the first session before committing to future ones. It is beneficial to explain that if they should begin to experience the slightest indication of sliding back to old habits, it will be easier to address the issues promptly rather than to wait until they are fully reinvested in their negative patterns. At times, it will be helpful to remind your clients that it may have taken a lifetime to attain the condition in which they find themselves. Therefore, it may take more than one to two hours of therapy to reverse the damage.

CHAPTER 17

Submodalities

It is important to understand the existence and use of submodalities. These adjectives metaphorically describe and define the client's conscious or subconscious experience. Such conceptualizations might include words and phrases such as:

- Proximity: near, far, close by, to the right, left, above me, below, behind, in front
- Texture: rough, smooth, gritty, spiked
- Time: soon, quickly, rapid, slow, occasionally, constant
- Color: red, blue, dark, pastel, luminescent, light, pale, opalescent
- Shape: square, round, oval, amorphous, like a cloud
- Density: heavy, solid, light, translucent, opaque
- Element: metallic, liquid, sandy, membrane, fire, airy
- Temperature: hot, cold, lukewarm, cool, icy, frigid
- Size: bigger than me, size of a baseball, two-inch diameter, miniscule, tall
- Sensation: throbbing, pulsing, still, heavy, vacant, vibrant, falling
- Mechanics: clutching, grabbing, choking, squeezing, releasing, pushing
- Comparisons: different from, same as

This list is by no means complete. However, it does give you an idea of how to assist your client in discovering their perceptions of their life.

Once discovered, the submodalities give you a concise "object" to work with. The chapter on Object Imagery will demonstrate how submodalities assist the client in altering or removing said "object" from their energy field or imagination. Thus, their perception of the issue is altered, allowing the feelings and emotions around it to change or dissipate.

> **During a session, a client disclosed strong negative feelings concerning her two older brothers. As she was the youngest and smallest, her memories were of them picking on her and being mean. The client revealed that her inner picture of their relationship showed her being in a ditch while they loomed tall over her on either side. Whenever she tried to make a move, they would push her back down or get in her way. When she was encouraged to alter their relative positions, she imagined herself as taller than her brothers. She then stepped out of the ditch and moved beyond them without impediment. She expressed great relief and a sense of freedom at last.**

Discovering the Client's Submodalities

By asking nonleading questions, the hypnotherapist can gain greater understanding of the client's internal experience. This will be particularly helpfully when facilitating Object Imagery techniques or when eliciting information about the client's condition, perceptions, or emotions.

Questions may include:

- "If I were to feel exactly the way that you do, what would I notice?"
- "If that sensation had a shape and a color, what would it be?"
- "If there was a metaphorical mechanism that produced that sensation, what would it look like and how would it operate?"
- "If you were to draw a picture of your relationship with your father, describe to me what the picture would look like."
- "If there was an animated cartoon depicting this condition, what would you notice about it?"

Once the details of the internal view are brought to light, there is a greater understanding of the perceived relationship between people, objects, sensations, and events. This knowledge affords the client a better opportunity to manipulate or eliminate them, creating greater comfort, release, and healing.

Control Panel

A fascinating tool, the Control Panel is generally received by the client with amusement and delight. The Control Panel gives the client control over their submodalities in a manner that is at once tangible and entertaining.

This technique creates a visual, and possibly auditory and kinesthetic, structure, completely devised and controlled by the client, for the regulation of the intensities of various experiences.

Creating the Control Panel

The panel may be imagined in any way that suits the client. It may have a couple of switches, or it may combine switches, levers, dials, knobs, and anything else the client requires.

When guiding the client through the creation of their control panel, keep your language as nonleading as possible.

Sample Script for Creating a Control Panel

"As you close your eyes, relaxing and breathing, imagine before you a control panel. It can look like anything you choose. Some people imagine theirs to resemble the bridge on 'Star Trek's' Enterprise, while others create control panels in other variations.

"As you examine the control panel before you, you begin to discover many levers, switches, dials, or knobs. Each one corresponds to an emotion, a reaction, a behavior, or a sensation that you would like to be able to regulate. One lever may sharpen your eyesight, while another may reduce pain. One dial may increase or decrease the intensity of your sadness, while a switch may allow you to quickly fall asleep.

"Take a few moments, now, to examine and experiment with your control panel."

Once the client indicates that their control panel has been set up, they can use it anytime in the future, or it can be incorporated into your dialogue during other parts of your session. For instance, if they have created a dial that increases courage, this can be utilized when the client is revisiting difficult memories.

Take a few moments to create a control panel for yourself. Using it in your own life will reveal additional ways in which to powerfully incorporate this technique into your sessions with clients.

CHAPTER 18

Guided Imagery, Suggestions, and Metaphor

Guided Imagery

Guided imagery is a popular technique that can be used alone or in combination with other hypnosis tools. As the title suggests, it involves the use of imagination and visualization, which is introduced by one person, typically the therapist, to another, the subject. Guided imagery is also referred to as guided visualization. Self-help tapes are a popular example of the use of guided imagery.

Who Benefits?

Guided imagery is helpful for clients who seek:

• Relaxation
• The expansion of imagination
• Guidance from one technique to the next
• Guidance from one perspective or condition to the next

How Does It Help?

With guided imagery, the client imagines the stories, metaphors, or descriptions that are presented by the therapist. In doing so, they may be able to:

• Look at an aspect of life from a different perspective
• Gain experience that they would not have in the normal course of their life

• Receive a metaphor for healing without interference from the critical mind
• Exercise their imagination
• Segue from one technique to the next
• Give themselves permission to be imaginative
• Follow instructions passively

Examples of guided imagery are presented in the scripts for Progressive Relaxation Induction, the Hallway deepening, and in Suggestibility Tests, among other techniques.

A Guided Imagery Script

"As you sit comfortably in your chair, relaxing, allow your attention to turn inwards. Notice the pattern of your breathing and the rhythm of your heart, as they find their own comfortable, relaxed pace.

"I wonder if you can imagine sitting on a park bench. All around you are rolling green lawns. As you sit there, contemplating, you look down at your feet and notice a large, empty box sitting open. You quickly realize that this is a special box. You are aware that you can allow all your stress and negative emotions to simply flow into that box.

"Imagine how good it will feel to release all those emotions and feelings of stress. To just let go of them. So, gathering them up inside of you, you begin to pour them into the box. Letting go of all the emotions that you are ready to release. Just letting them go. You may be able to identify the source of some of those emotions; you may know exactly what they are. Other emotions you may simply choose to release, letting go, without really understanding their origin or content. Just knowing that it feels so good to let go and release. Feeling so good, letting it happen.

"Do not feel obligated to release any emotions that still have a purpose for you. You can release all the negative feelings that you desire.

"And now, having poured all those unwanted stresses and feelings into that box, imagine, if you will, closing the lid of the box. There is string available to tie the box securely. When you do so, balloons appear—bright, colorful, helium balloons—which you can attach to the string around the box. Imagine tying enough balloons to this box that it begins to lift off the ground. As it gently floats upwards, you give it a little push away from you.

"Now watch that box, with all its balloons, as it floats up into the sky, ever higher. Getting smaller and smaller as it floats up into the blue sky. Drifting away, as you break any energetic ties with that box and its contents. Watching the box as it floats high up into the sky and . . . finally becomes a speck, and disappears.

"Now, turn your attention back to yourself, sitting on the bench. So relaxed. Notice how good you feel, released and relaxed. Feel the clarity and the balance as you enjoy the park and the rolling green lawns.

"And bringing this good feeling with you now, as I count from one to five, returning here to this present moment, refreshed and relaxed. One, two, three, coming up, four, aware of this time and space, and five, fully alert and here in the present moment."

We use guided imagery whenever we are delivering metaphors, telling stories, or in any way creating an image for another person to visualize. All metaphors and stories contain imagery.

Suggestion Therapy

Historically, hypnotherapy consisted of guiding a client to a deep state of trance and then implanting suggestions that would create the healing, relief of pain, and behavior or

---

While suggestion therapy is very powerful, its results may vary if the fundamental issues have not been addressed and relieved.

---

perception changes that were desired. This, of course, contributed greatly to the misconception that hypnosis involves mind control.

A Metaphor to Illustrate

A habit or syndrome is like a weed. The gardener may mow it down, but because the roots are still in the ground, eventually it will sprout and grow again. Similarly, suggestion therapy may "mow down" the symptom, but if the initial sensitizing event has not been extracted, the problem may surface again after a while.

Some people report good results immediately after suggestive hypnosis and then notice the effects eventually wear off.

When to Use

Suggestion therapy is best used after all other therapies are administered. Certainly, the results will be questionable until after Secondary Gains and Parts Therapy have been successfully completed.

The exception to this rule would be when simply giving suggestions that the client remember what happened during the session, and other suggestions that have to do with their immediate state.

Formulating Effective Suggestions

Creating suggestions is a process that is both simple and complex. Once the formula is understood, the appropriate suggestions are easy to produce. However, the complexity arises in the discovery of the pertinent information for a given client and their particular presenting issue.

Begin by following this formula:

1. Define the presenting problem. This information may be extrapolated from the presession interview or through direct questioning of the client. Use the subject's vocabulary and style of expression in your suggestions to maintain rapport.

2. List the opposites. Find the opposite condition or feeling, and create a corresponding word or phrase that will be used in the construction of the suggestion.

3. Construct the suggestion. From the above list of opposites, construct phrases that will be embedded in sentences, stories, and metaphors.

Examples

Client's Words and Phrases	Opposite Words and Phrases	Suggestions
Unsure	Confident	I wonder if you will begin to sense your confidence growing now or by tomorrow.
Stressed out	Relaxed	As you feel the sup port of the chair against your back, you may discover how easy it is to relax.

Ingredients for Successful Suggestions

Suggestions, like affirmations, must contain the following:

- Acceptable information—If a woman who needs to lose eighty pounds is given the suggestion that she will look like Twiggy next month, her conscious and subconscious minds will reject that immediately. The subject will also reject any suggestion that is counter to their morals and valuesor beyond their ability to handle or comprehend.
- Realistic timeframe—Use words like "now," "in the days and weeks to come," and "within the week," for example. If you simply state that the pain will go away, it will, but maybe not until the client is deceased!
- Positive wording—The mind cannot comprehend the negative without first imagining it in the positive. In other words, if the client is told, "Don't smoke that cigarette," they have to imagine smoking, and then try to banish the thought. It will be counterproductive.

Embedded Commands

Suggestions gain even greater power when embedded in sentences in such a way that they no longer seem like suggestions. For example: "Life seems more pleasant when you are relaxed." "My mother always told me that your self-confidence is stronger when you feel appreciated." There are two embedded suggestions in the preceding so sentence. Do you see them?

It may take practice to really become comfortable formulating and delivering suggestions. Studying the formula and writing out possible suggestions will give you the confidence to use them with your clients. With time, you may be surprised how easy it is to incorporate suggestions into your client sessions without having to prepare them in advance. You will develop the ability to improvise with confidence.

Metaphor

A metaphor is a symbolic image meant to correlate to, or substitute for, something else. It is synonymous with a simile or an analogy. A metaphor consists of a descriptive story, while guided imagery, alone, may lack significant or relevant meaning to the client.

Metaphors are a time-tested method of delivering a message to the conscious mind through a nonresistant subconscious door. Throughout history, stories have been used to reinforce morals, teach historical lessons, and offer us experiences that we would not otherwise have. In hypnotherapy, it is known that the easiest way to deliver a healing message to the subconscious mind is to bypass the barriers of the conscious mind by couching it in a symbol-rich tale that correlates to the presenting issue.

What makes metaphors so powerful is that they do bypass the critical factor in our analytical minds or emotional and ego responses. While the conscious mind listens to the story, the subconscious searches for meaning and resolution. Metaphors allow the client to create their own change, facilitating new learning without encountering resistance.

> **The subconscious mind more readily accepts a hidden metaphorical message than a direct command.**

Using Therapeutic Metaphors

The perfect metaphor, which will gain the desired results, requires an amount of research. To make it specific to the client, the therapist will:

- Collect data from the client that makes the story resonate with them
- Be aware of preferences, fears, and phobias
- Create a story that has symbolic meaning and correlations to the issue
- Devise a resolution, and deliver it in symbolic terms

Metaphorical stories are most effective when they contain the three main sense elements—visual, auditory, and kinesthetic.

> **Metaphor always includes imagery, but imagery does not always include a metaphor.**

CHAPTER 19

Reverse Metaphor

As therapists, we understand that the subconscious mind is already aware of its needs. Because there is a communication barrier between the subconscious mind and the conscious mind, the subconscious mind generally delivers its message through aches, pains, health conditions, habits, dreams, emotions, and behaviors. In Reverse Metaphor therapy, the subconscious mind has the opportunity to send its personalized message to the conscious mind in a way that is more intelligible. With understanding of the message, the client is then capable of delivering a viable and acceptable solution.

Development of Reverse Metaphor

Through my years as a clinical hypnotherapist and practitioner of NLP, it was obvious that the client's subconscious mind was capable of creating an explicit and elegant metaphor to communicate its message. I began asking the client to make up a story, a metaphor, around the issue. The symbols and images, naturally, were specifically in harmony with the meaning of the message originating in their deepest mind and emotions. The problem, along with its path to resolution, was delivered with pinpoint accuracy.

At that time, I was unaware that this was an undocumented therapy technique. I named it the Reverse Metaphor and began teaching the technique in hypnotherapy classes and conferences in the U.S. and abroad.

The reason behind naming it Reverse Metaphor is to indicate the twist from the typical metaphor therapy. A metaphor, as we are taught traditionally, is a story that the hypnotherapist tells to the client to deliver a message to the subconscious mind, thereby creating conditions for healing. I tagged the word "reverse" onto it to indicate that, in this case, the subconscious mind is delivering the story to the conscious mind, so that it can respond with the desired or necessary actions.

> **The subconscious mind eloquently reveals its desires and needs through Reverse Metaphor.**

When to Use Reverse Metaphor

Reverse Metaphor may prove to be one of the easiest tools you will have at your disposal in the therapeutic session. Once you become familiar with the methods and its diverse uses, you may find yourself resorting to it frequently, and in a wide range of circumstances.

It can easily be used in place of an induction technique. Simply ask the client to sit back, relax, close their eyes, and breathe. Then proceed with Reverse Metaphor as described below.

It is the most resourceful tool available when the client appears to be "stuck" or when their analytical mind just will not give up control or hypervigilance.

The Reverse Metaphor will fire up the imagination when you are seeking solutions beyond the client's normal range of ideas, experiencing difficulties eliciting information through other techniques, or encouraging clarity when the client has responded with "I don't know."

Prime Opportunities for Reverse Metaphor

A few of the many opportunities to utilize the Reverse Metaphor technique include:

- When unsure where to start with a client
- When seeking to discover the most important issue to address, out of a list the client has delivered
- When feeling less than resourceful in choosing the best tool for the presenting issue
- When the client needs more choices or ideas for resolutions to their issues
- When searching for the source of chronic illness, pain, and so forth

- When the client has an issue that they are not comfortable revealing in direct language
- When there is an extra ten to twenty minutes in your session to fill with productive work

Reverse Metaphor can be used entirely on its own, taking up the whole session.

Moreover, it can be used in combination with many other tools. For instance, it can be used in the middle of Parts Therapy, allowing one of the parts to create a Reverse Metaphor to reveal its perspective in a different manner. It can be applied during Object Imagery, which is already a use of metaphor. The "object" can tell a metaphorical story of its origins and its suggestions for the path of recovery.

The Techniques of Reverse Metaphor

It is important—in fact, vital—to remain nonleading and client centered while facilitating a Reverse Metaphor. The images, experience, and wisdom discovered and deciphered must all come from the client.

Refrain from attempting any therapy, any interjection whatsoever, during the storytelling and interpretation phases of the technique. Therapy and alterations will be applied at the conclusion of the technique.

Maintain fastidious notes (as always), transcribing all nouns and relevant verbs. Consider listing each item in a column for easier reference at the conclusion of the story. Interpretations can then be written next to the symbol.

Reverse Metaphor as Induction

"Sitting back comfortably, eyes closed, breathing naturally. I wonder if you can imagine a ball of light at your feet, glistening, shining, and radiating. And as that ball of light begins to move up across your body, it begins to gather up the perceptions and sensations. As it moves cross your legs, and your lap. Moving across your torso, your throat, and right on up into the center of your forehead.

"As this area of your forehead begins to energize, it strengthens the connections between your conscious and subconscious minds. This allows the subconscious mind to communicate more fully with the conscious mind, delivering its desires, concerns, and messages.

"Now, I would like to ask the subconscious mind to create for us a story, a metaphor, that will help us to understand its message. We may not know where the story begins or ends, or what happens in between, simply allowing it to unfold before us as we proceed through the story.

"To begin this process, imagine a hallway stretching out before you. This hallway can look like anything you choose. And as you begin to move down along this hallway, you begin to notice the texture of the floor covering beneath your feet, and the color of the walls. There are doorways along this hall. Each one leading to information, metaphors, that will help us to understand the message of the subconscious mind.

"As I count from three to one, you will find yourself in front of one of these doors. Three, two, one. How would you describe the door where you are standing?

"Are you ready to step through this door?" (Pause for affirmative client response.)

"Open the door and step through. Do you find yourself indoors or outdoors?"

From here, simply proceed with nonleading questions that will allow the client to discover the details of this story.

When they have completed that, start at the beginning of the story and name each scene, idea, noun, and verb they used. Ask them what each of these words would symbolize in their present life. The wording used could be similar to this:

"At the beginning of the story you mentioned you were in a _____. If that were a metaphor for something that is going on in your life here, what would that mean to you?"

Continue with this line of questioning concerning each item, throughout the metaphor.

Useful Tips

- If the client begins to tell you a memory, an experience, instead of a metaphor, gently acknowledge that it is a remembered event, and ask them to start again. Sometimes it helps to suggest they tell a story, as though they were telling a bedtime story to a child.
- It is typically rather evident when the client reaches the end of the

story. Simply keep asking, "Is there anything else?" until he or she says no.

• Sometimes the metaphor is self-evident and each of the items will not need to be examined for meaning. If this is the case, ask them what the story, as a whole, means to them and what they have learned from it.

• If the client states they do not know what the symbol means, ask them to guess. The subconscious mind knows what the symbol means, so a part of the client already does know. Inhibitions, or the fear of being wrong, may be removed by asking them to guess.

• Reverse Metaphor techniques can successfully be used in dream interpretation. Ask the client to tell you the dream three times, adding more and more information with each telling. Then go through the dream, as with Reverse Metaphor, to decipher the meanings of the symbols.

The Reverse Metaphor will be the therapy tool of choice when you are working with clients who are resistant or overly analytical. This method will enhance your client's comfort in using their imagination.

> **Frequently, clients reveal the details of their plight for the first time ever through Reverse Metaphor.**

By using the Reverse Metaphor, you will also give your clients a sense of protection when they are disclosing sensitive or embarrassing issues, such as those relating to abuse and sexuality. When the process is complete, they feel more comfortable disclosing the true-life story. This may be due to the relief they experience in disclosing the metaphor, which allows a part of them to feel they have already released the information. Occasionally, a client will admit they are revealing secrets that they have never told to anyone before. It is an honor to receive their trust. It is heartwarming to witness their lifelong burdens lifted and released. These are rich rewards for our work as hypnotherapists.

CHAPTER 20

Regression Therapy

Regression refers to the facilitation of remembering the past. Strictly speaking, it entails clients actually feeling themselves to be younger and perhaps smaller. The client may also achieve the observation of the memories from the perspective of a third party, or what is termed "dissociated."

Revealing Memories

The purpose of this exercise would include retrieval of memories, clarification of events and feelings, discovery of the root cause of some malady or habit, and the facilitation of therapy while in the regressed state to alter the perception of those events and their long-term impact on the client. Hypnosis takes us to the memories, while the facilitation of changes would require other techniques, such as those detailed later in this book.

Regression can also allow a client to recapture resources that they have somehow left behind or forgotten. These may include innocence, trust, bravery, confidence, self-esteem, joy, or a sense of safety. Reclaiming these characteristics will be addressed in detail in the chapter on Personality Part Retrieval. Regression will be utilized when facilitating Inner Child work, also detailed in a later chapter.

Imagination, Memory, and the Facts

Hypnosis may allow the client to reveal information that they previously were, or in other circumstances would be, more reserved in sharing. Relaxation and rapport may soften the client's boundaries on revealing such information. This may also lead to the client feeling freer to embellish information of which they previously felt unsure.

As imagination is a natural ingredient in the hypnotherapy session, boundaries between reality and fantasy may soften. This goes both ways—the client thinking that real memories may actually be fantasy or concluding that what they have imagined may be factual. Hypnotic states may also provide the opportunity for fantasy and reality to be intertwined.

Because the hypnotic state allows the subject to experience increased suggestibility, it is vital for the hypnotherapist to ask neutral questions, use language that in no way contaminates the memories of the client, and avoid using even the most subtle cues. Contamination of the session may occur intentionally or unintentionally, even with the greatest care.

Using Neutral Language

The following are good examples of neutral, nonleading statements and questions that can freely be used in a regression session:

Take me back to a time . . .	Tell me about the last time . . .
What are you experiencing?	What do you notice?
What happens next?	And then what?
What is that experience for you?	What does that mean to you?
Describe what you are observing.	What else do you notice?

Avoid the use of the words "see" and "hear." Only use specific senses when the client has already indicated that they are seeing or hearing something. If the subject is an auditory or kinesthetic person, and the question is expressed, "What do you see?" they may think that they are failing in the session. There is a risk of breaking rapport.

> **Hypnosis does not guarantee the truth; it is not truth serum.**

It is possible for clients to lie or intentionally distort the truth while under hypnosis. Likewise, hypnosis does not make a client omniscient. It is possible the client misses, or remains unaware of, valuable information because it falls outside their philosophy or religious beliefs or they refuse to face those facts at present.

Positive Regression

Similar to regression, positive regression allows the client to return to a time when they had a specific desirable trait or resource. By recalling and reinforcing that trait, they may use it while treading into more negatively charged memories or while anticipating frightening future events.

A script for a positive regression may sound like this:

"As you continue to relax, breathing, allow your mind to drift back,

Positive regression is also a way to end a session with a pleasant mindset.

back to a time when you remember being happy. That's right. Going to a memory of a time when you felt life was good and you were joyful. Very good. And as you go back to that time, to that pleasant and wonderful time, begin to tell me about that event, as you experience it now."

As they reach the pinnacle moment of that experience of happiness, you will want to anchor those sensations. Refer to the chapter on anchoring for a complete description of this technique.

Call upon positive regression to revivify a happier time in the client's life. When a person is suffering from acute depression, or finds themselves in the midst of turmoil and tragedy, it is easy to lose sight of the fact that there have been pleasant, joyful moments in life. By accessing those memories of happiness, the client is encouraged to seek a balanced perspective in their otherwise dreary situation or condition.

Achieving Regression

Again, the use of regression is typically just a vehicle to achieve the memory of those earlier years. Two language patterns make this journey swift and effortless.

Affect Bridge—The Affect Bridge connects events and experiences through their common affects, or emotions. "Take me to the last time you felt . . ." When they have told you about the most recent episode, continue, "Now take me to the previous time you felt . . ." Continue in this manner until there are no previous correlating events. At this point, it is typical for the client to have an abreaction.

Somatic Bridge—The Somatic Bridge connects events and experiences through their common somatic indices, or physical attributes—typically pain or bouts of illness. The language is the same: "Take me to the last time you experienced . . ." When they have told you about the most recent episode, continue, "Now take me to the previous time you experienced . . . " Continue in this manner until there are no previous experiences to report. Again, there may be an abreaction at this point.

In each case, we term this as returning to root cause, or to the initial sensitizing event. While moving backwards in time towards that initial event, we are merely collecting data. The client is recounting their personal perspective of history as it relates to their life and the presenting problem. No therapy techniques are being administered beyond the very potent one of being a good listener. Simply allow the stories to unfold.

There will be a part of their subconscious mind that is drawing numerous conclusions, noticing patterns, and having "ah-ha" experiences. These will be revealed shortly. For now, though, your responsibility is to listen and guide the client, noninvasively, through their memories.

It is highly likely that the client will experience an abreaction when they arrive at the initial sensitizing event. Remember that when your client spontaneously abreacts, they are already going into a trance state. For instance, if your client is telling you about a recent argument with their spouse and begins to cry, they are entering a natural trance state. Use this opportunity to move right into the session. Gently suggest the following:

"I notice that you are connecting with your emotions around this issue. Why don't you just sit back and close your eyes. That's right. Now continue telling me that story."

This is so much more elegant and client centered than listening to their story, drying their tears, going through a formal induction, and then requesting that they tell you the story all over again. Moving harmoniously with them in the moment saves so much time and energy.

Is It Real?

The truthfulness of the memory is not as vital a point as one might expect. What is of the utmost importance is the impact created by the client's perspective of these events.

Quantum physics has demonstrated that very little of what we perceive as the physical world has anything to do with reality. The field of psychology now confirms that every experience we have is filtered through the "colored glasses" of our emotions, family of origin issues, ethnic and cultural background, environment, education, and more.

When we observe our memories, or listen to those of our clients, we are actually witnessing the nature of those filters.

A college student came to the office and revealed that since the age of eleven she was certain that her father did not love her. During the intake, she disclosed that her parents had divorced during that year and her father had moved away. Although he continued to visit and give support, she was convinced that in his heart he did not love her. Through regression work, she was able to gain a greater understanding of their relationship. She discovered that in fact he did love her and had shown it throughout their relationship. He simply could not stay married to her mother. Upon emerging, she excitedly stated that she was immediately going to contact her father and strengthen their bonds.

Forensic Hypnosis

If a client seeks discovery of information that will assist them in a lawsuit, it would be wise to refer them to a qualified forensic hypnotherapist. Stringent criteria must be met for the extracted information to be valid in a court of law. You would be doing a great disservice to all parties involved, and to justice, should this type of case be handled improperly.

Can We Change the Past?

There may or may not be ways to change the past to a degree. What is more important is that we can change our perceptions of it. In doing so, we can adjust our emotional and subconscious responses into healthier ones. This allows us to alter the nature of the filters that define our experience of reality in the present and into the future.

A large part of the fascinating information we will be discussing in this book has to do with the very techniques that will allow those changes to be made.

CHAPTER 21

Secondary Gains

It is fascinating that everything we choose to do has a secondary gain involved. By secondary gains, we mean there is a benefit that is derived from whatever behavior or choice we make, no matter how negative or self-sabotaging it appears to be.

As these secondary gains are uncovered, you and your client will become more fully apprised of any motives, whether hidden or overt, that will sabotage efforts towards healing. Therefore, it is strongly advised to uncover these secondary gains early in your work with a client, returning to this tool each time a new topic or issue is addressed.

When to Use Secondary Gains

This is a "must-use" technique when working on issues of self-sabotage, particularly in cases of chronic illness, weight retention, smoking, addictions, and abusive relationships.

Frequently when you begin the session with secondary gains, it will lead very gracefully into Parts Therapy. By doing this, the hypnotherapist could bypass using formal inductions. After working through these two techniques, the client is typically in full trance.

Setting Up Secondary Gains

The questions may be posed in a number of ways, yet all sets consist of four questions. You are seeking the positive and negative aspects of having the presenting condition and the positive and negative aspects of not having the condition.

Here are a few ways that the questions may be posed. Choose whichever group best suits the situation.

Set 1

What does having (this condition) allow you to do?
What does having (this condition) prevent you from doing?
What would not having (this condition) allow you to do?
What would not having (this condition) prevent you from doing?

Set 2

In what way is (this behavior) a benefit to your life?
In what way is (this behavior) a detriment to your life?
In what way would not doing (this behavior) be a benefit to your life?
In what way would not doing (this behavior) be a detriment to your life?

Set 3

How is (this condition/behavior) positive or supportive for your goals?
How is (this condition/behavior) negative or nonsupportive of your goals?
How would not having (this condition/behavior) be positive for your goals?
How would not having (this condition/behavior) be negative for your goals?

The Client's Experience

It is very easy for the questions to sound invasive and threatening. A client may be quite con-

> **It is important to ask the questions in a respectful and gentle manner.**

fused when asked how does staying in an abusive relationship benefit their life. However, there has to be some benefit or they would not continue to do so.

It is typical for the client to have an "ah-ha" experience with this technique. They have the opportunity to look at their issue from angles they have not previously explored. As simple as the questions appear to be, they are terrifically powerful in eliciting information, hidden motives, and the potential for sabotage.

Once the answers to the questions are discovered, the client will understand previously unrecognized information about him or herself, and the hypnotherapist will have a much clearer picture of how to proceed in the session with additional therapy techniques.

Case Study for Secondary Gains

Secondary Gains is a strong beginning point when working with clients who wish to lose weight. Observe the richness of information that comes from these questions. The technique naturally provides clues to the underlying issues that will have to be addressed in order for the client to be successful in any weight-loss program. Following are excerpts from a session:

ML: What does retaining the weight allow you to do?

Client: It keeps me from focusing on the issue of attractiveness. I can do a nominal job of getting dressed in the morning.

ML: What does retaining the weight prevent you from doing?

Client: It prevents me from attracting handsome men who care about looks. The men who will like me will appreciate intelligence and drive. It also prevents me from dealing with rejection from men who I've been attracted to. The weight also self-perpetuates. I'm not as physically active and therefore it is harder to lose. It prevents me from having an exciting sex life. I don't feel attractive and I don't initiate intimacy. It also prevents me from enjoying clothes shopping and having as much energy as I could have.

ML: What would losing the weight allow you to do?

Client: It would change how I see myself. I would feel more like myself. I could do things I enjoy, like rollerblading. I would enjoy dressing attractively. I would feel more in my body. More grounded. Going up and down stairs would be easier. I would feel younger, more vital, and not sluggish.

ML: What would losing the weight prevent you from doing?

Client: I would have to quit hiding. I have fear of a structured life. It would mean that I would have to give up the foods that I like.

From this dialogue, the facilitator becomes aware of several underlying issues that will have to be resolved before success can be expected from any weight-loss program. From these answers, a strategy for therapy can be developed.

While studying Parts Therapy in the next chapter, you will surely see the elegant role that secondary gains will play in preparing both the hypnotherapist and the client for that technique.

CHAPTER 22

Parts Therapy

Also known as Ego States Therapy, Parts Therapy is one of the most versatile tools available.

How many times do we say, "Part of me wants to do this, and another part of me doesn't"? Life is filled with decisions and quandaries that create inner turmoil, confusion, and conflict. Parts Therapy is just the tool to use!

Our personalities are comprised of a multitude of aspects. Some parts are healthy ones that have adapted to life's stresses in useful, protective, or socially acceptable ways. Other parts may prove to be more difficult, creating blocks to our growth, self-sabotaging behaviors, violence, rage, and chronic illness. Some parts may have developed so fully and separately from the main personality that the person is declared to have multiple-personality disorder.

Regardless of the extent of separation, or whether they contribute positively or negatively to the person's life, all parts included in the consciousness of the individual think that they are doing the best that they can for the survival of the individual.

Using Parts Therapy

The usefulness of Parts Therapy is guaranteed because the technique can be applied to most presenting issues, is easy to use, and can be done almost anywhere, anytime, without prior trance induction. By simply setting up the therapy, the person falls deeper and deeper into trance as the therapy proceeds. Use Parts Therapy in cases of:

- Indecision
- Inner conflict
- Self-sabotage
- Hearing voices
- Unexplained, unwanted behaviors
- Posttraumatic stress disorder
- Blocks to creativity, healing, and change
- Chronic illness and pain
- Unexplained illness and pain
- Resistance to the therapy process
- Removing the critical factor or the "Analytical Imp"

What is interesting about this is that each and every client will come into the office suffering from some type of issue that could be well served, if not alleviated altogether, through the use of Parts Therapy. There is a part of them that wants to heal and another part that has resisted doing it on their own—or they would not have needed to pay you for your services!

When a hypnotherapist proceeds with Parts Therapy, it is imperative to remain respectful and client centered. Each part is doing its best to assist the client even if its efforts appear counterproductive. When the part senses hostility towards it, or feels threatened by the hypnotherapist or the process, it will be less inclined to consider options for change and growth. It is more likely to cooperate if it senses that its efforts have been appreciated and that, together, you will all be seeking an even more important, and successful, way for the part to operate.

Steps in Setting Up Parts Therapy

1. Determine the distinct polarity of the issue, eliciting two parts.
2. Direct the parts to each migrate to one of the client's hands, completely separating.
3. Ask the client to "go into" one of the hands, completely, becoming fully identified with only that part.
4. Ask that part to verbalize its position in the matter, without interference from the other part. Allow it to speak, uninterrupted until finished.
5. Move to the other part, asking it to verbalize its position, just as above.
6. Alternate between hands, until they have reached an agreement to cooperate with each other. Ask the client to verbalize that agreement.

7. Determine whether any other part objects to the agreement.
8. Integrate the two parts.

Example of Parts Therapy

An induction may be administered first, or simply start with secondary gains. Then proceed with the following dialogue:

"Is it true for you that there is a part of you that would like to _____ and another part of you that resists or sabotages that effort?"

Fill in the appropriate language pertinent to the issues that the client has presented to you. Always open the therapy by posing this type of question. Frequently the wording you use is not exactly how the client would state it. Do not proceed until the client has concurred with the exact labeling of the two parts.

"Now, begin to imagine that these two parts of you are completely separated, so distinctly that you could put all of the part that wants to _____ on one of your hands, and all of the part that resists that on the other hand.

"And as you do so, which hand contains the part of you that wants to _____?

"And the other hand, your [right or left] hand, holds all of the part that resists that. Is that correct?

"Continue to completely separate those two parts of you so that they in no way intersect. And when you have done that, allow yourself to go into the _____ side, the side that wants to _____.

"Allow this side to express whatever it has to say about its position, its goals and desires—without any interruption whatsoever from the other side. What would it have to say?

"Is there anything else that it would like to say?

"Anything else?

"OK and now, come out of that side, and all the way over to the other side, the side that wants to _____. And without any interruption from the other side, what does it have to say about its position?

"Is there anything else that it would like to say?

"Anything else?

"OK . . . come back over to the _____ side, and what would it have to say about what it just heard?

"Anything else?

"OK. Now, come back over to the _____ side. What would it have to say about what it just heard?

"Anything else?

"Coming back over to the _____ side, what does this side have to say now?

"Anything else?

"Coming back over to the _____ side, what does this side have to say now?

"Anything else?

"And what does it feel like, being on this side?

"Moving back to the other side, what does it feel like being on this side?"

Continue this line of questioning until the two sides have fully expressed themselves and have begun to move closer together in resolving their differences.

Typically, the side that has been offering resistance to the positive direction that the client desires begins to weaken and agree with the healthier side. When this occurs, you may continue as follows.

"Have these two sides come to an agreement to work together to further your goals?" (Wait for a yes. If the response is no, continue the dialogue until such an agreement can be reached.)

"Tell me what the agreement is that you have made between you." (Always have the client state the agreement. Articulating it will clarify it in their mind and apprise you of exactly what they are agreeing to do.)

"Is that agreeable to both sides?

"Is there any other part that would disagree with this arrangement?" (Occasionally, another part has additional concerns. If there is such a part, continue this line of dialogue with the two agreeing sides on one hand now and the opposing part on the other hand. Typically, there is no further disagreement.)

"Now, bringing your hands together, in agreement, slowly, as these two parts fully integrate. Becoming one. Agreeing to work together, as one, for the furtherance of these goals. Holistically. Now bringing these integrated parts into your body . . . your heart . . . your very soul. Working together with the highest purpose that is best for the entire being. That's right. Very good.

"How does that feel now?"

Always integrate the parts before closing the session. Be sure to check with the client as to their feelings—both emotionally and physically. This allows them the opportunity to express anything that they feel may have been left undone. However, the client nearly always expresses amazement at the wonderful, unified feeling that they have, and the resolve to achieve their desired goals without hindrance from the previously resistant part.

Pointers for Successful Application of Parts Therapy

- There will only be two parts involved. If it appears that there are three or more parts involved, rethink the problem. Perhaps you are including more than one problem. For example, the client expresses to the hypnotherapist that they are in a quandary about whether to get married or not, and there is an additional concern about whether to finish college. The client may think that the issues are intertwined and, in some way, they may be. However, the job of a hypnotherapist is to separate the issues into clear components. By working on the singular problem of one part wanting to get married and the other part resisting marriage, the subject of college may end up aligning with one of those sides. If it does not end up on one side of this issue, then it needs to be dealt with as a separate problem.
- Always ask the client if they agree to the wording of the identity of each side. Even with the information gained during your presession discussion, the labels used for each side may not be in precisely the terms that resonate with the client. Guide them in discovering the correct wording, as the terms must express the client properly.
- Keep your language as noninvasive and nonleading as possible. Avoid putting words or ideas into the client's experience. We cannot assume to know what they are thinking and feeling, or how the best outcome will be developed.
- Allow each side to fully express itself. Part of the client's dilemma has been that the issues are entangled in their mind, or in their emotions. Neither part has ever been allowed to fully express itself without being put down, interrupted, or dismissed. By respectfully allowing both sides to express themselves fully, they can achieve satisfaction and begin to feel secure about working out a compromise.
- During the presession talk, the client will be expressing the two sides of the issue. It will become apparent to the sensitive hypnotherapist

which side should be expressed first when beginning the therapy. If the client has begun to get emotional while talking about one side of the issue, that would be the side to start with. The client is already resonating with that side and beginning abreaction. To switch, and ask the other side to express its concerns first, would risk being quite awkward or disconcerting, and possibly breaking rapport. If there is no real dominant side at the beginning of the Parts Therapy, the hypnotherapist has the option of choosing a side to begin with, or asking the client to make the choice.

• After each part has expressed itself a couple of times, and perhaps has ceased to add new information during its turn, it would be advantageous to ask how that side feels, or ask the client how they feel when they are in that side. Typically, the positive goal-oriented side will be light, optimistic, and ready to change and grow. The resistant side will frequently feel darker, heavier, depressed, fearful, and so forth. Bringing the client's attention to the difference in the feelings may help to clarify their decisions and determine the course of action.

• It is oftentimes advisable and productive to do other types of therapy on one of the parts—most particularly the resistant part. This need becomes obvious when the part has trouble moving off its position, for whatever reason. Useful therapies to resolve this quandary may include Outcomes, Inner Child work, or Object Imagery addressed to this one part.

• Always complete the session with integration. The last thing a hypnotherapist wants to do is to create multiple-personality disorders or even the slightest division of the personality. If the session has to be closed before an agreement is reached between the two parts, have them agree to disagree, or come to some interim agreement, requesting that the subconscious and conscious minds continue to work on the agreement until the next appointment.

Always Integrate the Parts

To effectively integrate the parts, the hypnotherapist can use the following guideline script:

"Now that these two parts of you have come to a satisfactory agreement as to their cooperation with each other in the furtherance of the goal of _____, I invite them to come together, physically, slowly, as these two parts integrate, completely. Coming together, in a clasp, in unison, agreeing [the

client's hands moving together]. That's right. Integrating, one goal, one direction. Working together. Feeling so powerful, whole, unified. That's right. And now, bringing that unification into your body, your mind, your heart, and your very soul. That's right. Experiencing the wholeness, the oneness, fully integrated. And how do you feel now?"

Most clients respond that it is an exhilarating experience. They find resolution to their conflicts and gain conviction to move ahead energetically and wholeheartedly towards their goals.

Avoid Critical Problems

Beware of certain pitfalls. Some hypnotherapists go so far as to give names to the parts, or to ask the part to give itself a name. The benefit of this practice is questionable. It tends to create a greater identity for the part rather than moving it closer to integrating smoothly with the main personality. By simply putting the part on one hand or another, the hypnotherapist can continue to distinguish one from the other without contributing more energy to its division.

Creating stronger identity for the part can enhance its separateness from the main personality. If done incorrectly, or if the integration process is not completed successfully at the end of the session, could this lead to greater possibilities of encouraging multiple-personality disorder?

If the part comes forth and declares a separate name, it can be used; however, this may also indicate that a client referral to a qualified psychiatrist may be in order.

Parts Therapy has proven to be an extraordinary and versatile technique that produces rapid and lasting resolution for problems both large and small.

**A minor child was brought in to the office by his parents.
He had been diagnosed with obsessive/compulsive behaviors.
The parents were concerned about the effects of placing him on
medication. Their medical specialist agreed that hypnotherapy
might alleviate the condition in a rapid, drug-free fashion. In
thirteen sessions, over a period of less than six months, all the
signs of the disorder had receded. The repeated use of Parts
Therapy, along with other techniques presented in this book,
created this swift return to normal life for this young man.**

CHAPTER 23

Object Imagery

Easy to use, Object Imagery may take place as an induction, in the midst of other techniques, or as the sole therapy for the session. Based on submodalities, this method uses the imagination to describe an object that is creating the discomfort—whether it is physical, emotional, or mental.

Object Imagery is an appropriate tool when the client is experiencing:

• Physical pain, temporary or chronic
• Symptoms of illness
• Emotional pain
• Abreaction
• Mental block
• Fear

Abreaction Can Replace Induction

It is not necessary to induce trance before beginning Object Imagery; however, it may enhance the early part of the therapy. While the client is cooperating with the technique, they are easing deeper and deeper into trance naturally.

When a client begins describing a pain or emotion that they are experiencing, or if they begin to abreact while discussing their issues for the session, it is easy to quickly and elegantly move right into Object Imagery. Simply ask them to sit back and relax, close their eyes, and begin describing the pain or emotion. Follow the steps for Object Imagery as they are listed below.

Indications for Object Imagery

Even without an emotional eruption, when a client begins a conversation about their experiences and uses terms such as those listed below, Object Imagery is a natural technique to instigate immediately.

- My relationship is like a ball and chain around my ankle.
- My job is like a weight on my shoulders.
- My mind goes blank whenever I try to write my book.
- My body freezes up whenever I get ready to take a test.
- My heart feels like a big black void.
- My troubles are hanging over my head.
- I feel like someone is choking me.
- I'm tripping over myself.
- My hands are tied.

The client has naturally begun to verbalize their internal pictures, so why not continue their train of thought in a productive manner. Even if the client has not expressed it in those terms, such as describing an internal picture, and even if you are in midsession with a client, the seasoned hypnotherapist can easily set up Object Imagery in the appropriate places.

To do so, simply ask the client what they are experiencing. Elicit the details of the physical sensations. You are looking for words like sharp, dull, throbbing, heavy, etc. Again, simply move straight into Object Imagery.

Translating Experiences into Metaphors

Frequently people are mildly to severely disconnected, or dissociated, from their physical functions and sensations. Therefore, the goal is to have the client become thoroughly aware of what is actually going on in their body.

If the client is having a difficult time articulating their experience, it may be helpful to ask them some questions, such as: "If I were to experience this sensation, how would I know whether it is exactly as you are experiencing it? What would I be noticing?"

Once they have described what they are experiencing, in detail, proceed by guiding the client into creating an imaginary object, a metaphor, that could represent this feeling or process they are experiencing.

The reason for having the client translate their sensation or feeling into a metaphorical image is to make it more concrete. In this way, they will be able to communicate with it, manipulate it, and perhaps eliminate it.

Trying to do the same things with a pain or emotion may be too "slippery" or amorphous. Having something solid to focus on gives them something to work with that is more tangible.

To achieve the goal of creating the object, questions such as the following could be used:

- "If this sensation were an object, something with a shape and a color, what would it be?"
- "If this pain had a shape and a color, what would you imagine it to be?"
- "If what you are experiencing had a shape and a color, or if it were an imaginary process that you could observe, how would you describe it?"

Typical responses are:

- A gray knot that has a death-grip on my stomach
- A black void in the middle of my chest
- A stone wall all around me
- A knife stabbing me
- A fountain welling up from my heart to my throat

Client responses will be as plentiful and varied as the experiences that have produced them. In order to stay immersed in the process with your client, it is advisable to determine the location, size, color, function, and any other information that you need in order to fully understand the object and how it operates.

Determine the Message

Once these have been established, you may begin a line of questioning to determine how to proceed in the best interests of your client. Some objects simply need to be heard, to have their message delivered. Some objects need to be manipulated, morphed, or eliminated.

However, before any changes take place, it is a good idea to assist the client in discovering the wisdom and lessons that this object is bringing to the client. No matter how destructive or obtrusive this object has appeared to be, it has been there because it has served an important purpose. It may provide important learning and growth.

In order to accomplish this, the hypnotherapist may proceed as follows:

"There is a part of your subconscious mind that knows exactly how to telepathically communicate with that object. If you could do so, how would that object describe its purpose?

"If the part of your subconscious mind that has created this object had a message for you, what would it tell you?

"In what way does this object feel or think that it has been functioning in service to your higher good?

"I wonder what wisdom could be shared by that part of your subconscious mind that has created this object.

"What could you learn from it, or what have you learned by having it there? In what way has it served you well?"

> **Typically, the part of the higher self that has created this object is protecting or in some way operating for the benefit of the client.**

Soliciting the Help of the Part

At this point, you may want to deliver a metaphor that will resonate with and provide understanding for the part. It goes like this:

"Sometimes our minds are like computers. Over time, we acquire certain programs that help us in our work and function very successfully. Later we find that our needs change and a program has become somewhat outdated. Perhaps there are ways to update the program so that it performs its function with even more successful results. In the same way, over time some of our behaviors and beliefs need to be updated so they are more in keeping with our maturity levels, or aligned with the changing situations or goals that we have in our lives. This part of the subconscious mind that has produced this object may be experiencing curiosity about exploring new ways of operating, so that it can serve an even more important function and achieve greater success in its efforts. Would you be willing to explore those possibilities?"

By stating this proposal in a way that gives respect to the part that has produced the object, a way that is nonthreatening, it is typical to get the approval, if not enthusiastic support, from that part in the process of discovering and implementing positive change. At times, the part may hesitate or be fearful of any changes. If this occurs, nurture the part and continue to find out what its concerns are and in what way they can be satisfied. Eventually, the part will agree to cooperate, if this step is presented properly. After all, its sole purpose in the first place was for the safety, survival, and happiness of the client.

If the object is showing resistance, consider resorting to separate therapeutic techniques, such as Outcome-based therapies, Inner Child work,

Regression, or even a tangential Parts Therapy. (See other chapters for the procedures for these techniques.)

Creating Resolution

Once the part has agreed to make the changes, begin exploring, with the client and the part, how they would like to see the transformation take place. You may ask one of the following questions:

- "In what way would you like to see this resolved?"
- "How could this object be transformed in a way that would allow you to achieve your goals, and at the same time satisfy this part of you?"
- "In what way could we change the shape and the color of this object so that it is more comfortable for you?"

Always allow the client to determine how they want this object, or this part, to change. Also, allow them to determine how rapidly the changes will take place. These questions generally elicit responses ranging from simply chang- ing the color or size of the object (the submodalities) to blowing the thing up. Some changes happen easily as the request to do so is made, or by the client using their imagination to visualize the changes. Other objects (parts) are more obstinate and are reluctant, or refuse, to change or be removed. If so, it is correct to suspect that there is still a part of the client that finds the object's purpose to be useful or comforting—even if it truly is self-defeating.

If the client has difficulty in removing the unwanted object, it may be a good idea to apply secondary gains to determine the remaining benefits that are derived from this object or part.

Replacements

Once the object is improved upon or removed, the hypnotherapist can ask the client to describe what is remaining in that location now. Sometimes there is an energetic residue, hole, or raw wound of some sort. Complete the healing with another visualization as follows:

"What do you notice in that area now? Is there anything else that needs to take place there? Is there further healing to do to complete this process . . . some energy, light, or other salve that could be applied?"

Some clients have chosen to fill the area with love, light, gemstones, energy, colors, flowers, feathers, a positive word, etc. Again, it is up to the client to choose what is appropriate for them. Once they have filled that area, or in some way completed the healing, you may proceed.

"Is there anything else that needs to be done? How is that area feeling now? Is there anything else that you notice happening in that area?"

From here, loop back to the original issue to find out what has now shifted in their perception of the issue and their emotions surrounding it. Ask for any other comments that the client would want to make.

Summary of the Technique

Use the following steps to set up Object Imagery:

1. The client describes the physical sensation.
2. The client translates the physical sensation into an object or process.
3. The client describes the function of the object or process.
4. Discover the inherent wisdom or lessons learned from having the object.
5. Determine what the client wants to do with it—maintain, alter, or discard it.
6. Facilitate that goal.
7. If the object was discarded, heal or fill the remaining space.
8. Ask the client if anything else needs to be done regarding this.
9. If so, facilitate it. If not, break state, talking about other things.
10. Focus again on that area and do an environment check. Is it still clear?

Object Imagery may substitute for a formal induction or be used in the midst of other therapy techniques. It is easy to apply during Regression or Parts Therapy, for example. Translating emotional or physical feelings into a metaphorical object allows the sensations to become more tangible and available for manipulation or elimination. This leads to easier, more rapid healing.

Practice Object Imagery on yourself. Notice your own internal images of pains or emotions. How can you change your experience of them by changing the shapes and colors of the images?

CHAPTER 24

Ideosensory and
Ideomotor Signals

Using Ideosensory and Ideomotor Signals allows the subconscious mind to bypass the critical factor, the analytical or opinionated mind, to deliver its message. Both methods use subconscious responses to yes and no questions. The difference between the two techniques is simply the manner in which the response is delivered.

Ideosensory Responses

When there is a somatic aspect (a pain or illness), or an emotional aspect (such as sadness or depression), the physical sensations produced by the condition can be used to accomplish the communication. As in Parts Therapy, the manifested part may be isolated and addressed as "the part of you that creates this pain." That part of the subconscious mind that has produced the said sensation or emotion is encouraged, then, to communicate with the client's conscious mind, by strengthening or weakening the physical sensation as indications of yes and no responses.

An example of eliciting an Ideosensory Signal follows:

"I would like to ask that part of your subconscious mind that is producing this sensation if it would be willing to communicate with us, for the purpose of discovering the message that it has and increasing our ability to satisfy its true needs. In order to enhance our ability to communicate with it, we would like to suggest that it use this same sensation as a signal. By either increasing or decreasing the intensity of this sensation, we will establish the signal for a 'yes' or positive response to my questions, and a "no, n-o" or negative response.

"So, please, give us a signal, now, for a 'yes' or positive response." (Wait for a response, asking the client to share with you what they are experiencing.)

"Very good. Thank you. Now, please, give us a signal for a 'no, n-o' response." (Again, wait for the response.)

"Very good. Now, I wonder what signal you will use for 'I don't know or I am not ready to respond.'" (Again, wait for the corresponding signal.)

"Once again, please reconfirm your response for 'yes'. . . and reconfirm your response for 'no'. . . and reconfirm your response for 'I don't know or am not ready to respond.'" (Again, wait after each request for the appropriate responses.)

Ideomotor Signals

Another way to communicate with the subconscious mind is through Ideomotor Signals. Similar to the Ideosensory Signals, they use responses that have originated in the subconscious mind. The difference is that they are typically set up by using the fingers from the right and/or left hands for the yes and no responses. The drawback with this technique is that it provides more room for the client to manipulate the responses. In the case of Ideomotor Signals, it is imperative that the client is deeply in trance. The hypnotherapist must stay vigilant that the responses are not being contaminated by the client's analytical, critical thinking.

To set up the Ideomotor Signals, the hypnotherapist would begin in a similar fashion by saying:

"I would like to ask that part of your subconscious mind that is in charge of this behavior if it would be willing to communicate with us, for the purpose of discovering the message that it has and increasing our ability to satisfy its true needs. In order to enhance our ability to communicate with it, I would like to suggest that it use movements in the fingers of the right and left hands to indicate 'yes' and 'no, n-o' responses to the questions that I will be asking. So please, now, indicate a signal that you would like to use for a 'yes' response to my questions. (Pause for the response.) *Thank you. Please indicate a 'no, n-o' response to my questions.* (Pause for the response again.) *Thank you.*

"Additionally, please show us a response that will indicate, 'I don't know, or refuse to answer at this time.' (Pause for the response). *Thank you."*

Once while I was eliciting an Ideomotor response from a client, an isolated muscle over his left rib cage tensed up when he responded affirmatively, and it completely relaxed for a negative response. Another client had a muscle in her neck cramp tightly for yes and release for no.

Pointers for Ideosensory and Ideomotor Signals

- The movements of the fingers will typically be jerky, slow, and appear to be spontaneous rather than willfully produced.
- Test responses for verification. Once the responses are consistent, proceed with your line of questioning.
- It is advisable to spell out "no" because the subconscious mind can be extremely literal and could perhaps confuse "no" with "know."
- A deep level of trance is mandatory for this method to be accurate and successful.
- It is important to double-check the signals to make sure that they are consistent and that they weren't just random or an apparition of the client's imagination.
- If the signals given during the reconfirmation are different from the original signals, start over to determine the correct signals or to allow the client to identify the correct responses. It is possible that the client has mistaken the signal, as they may be learning this technique for the first time.
- Sometimes there is no substantial difference between the signals for yes and no. If the client is unable to distinguish them at all, continue working until two distinct signals are discovered. Alternatively, it may be wise to defer to an altogether different strategy.
- When the signals are too faint or excruciatingly painful, feel free to request that the subconscious mind turn up the volume or tone down the pain. It is fascinating to watch how the subconscious mind will actually follow that direction and make the requested changes.

By directing the subconscious to alter the submodality of the signal, such as turning up the volume or reducing the pain, the client has the opportunity to begin to learn a remarkable aspect of this pain. To wit: the manipulation of the intensity of this pain is within their control. Pain does not have to be a constant in their life and they may learn ways to alter it. There is hope!

Guidelines for Questions

Once the hypnotherapist has established the corresponding signals, the next step is to formulate sound questions. Be aware of the following guidelines:

- Remember that all questions must be asked as yes and no questions.
- Keep the questions simple. Remember that the subconscious mind, like the conscious mind, can become very confused by wordiness, stringed phrases, and convoluted questions.
- Formulate nonleading questions.
- Avoid mind reading and making assumptions.
- Avoid questions that could have several meanings or elicit confusing responses.
- Create questions with a timeframe when possible. For example: "Would this part be willing to make these changes now?"

If the parts are presenting themselves as a behavior, rather than a pain, Ideosensory Signals can still be established. Instead of using the intensity of the presenting pain, request that the subconscious mind choose an involuntary muscle, or some other bodily response, through which to communicate. It may choose to tense and release a muscle that the client cannot consciously control. Client responses have included flushing in the face and heat in the ears.

Ideosensory Signals are accurate responses because the client's conscious mind cannot interfere by interjecting its own interpretations or expectations.

Review for Facilitating Ideosensory and Ideomotor Signals

1. Determine the issue.
2. Induce a deep state of trance.
3. Allow the client to create a signal for "yes," "no," and "I can't or won't answer that." It may be the movement of separate fingers, involuntary fluctuations in tension of a muscle, or a change in the intensity of a pain they have.
4. Test the signals for accuracy.
5. Ask succinct questions appropriate to eliciting yes and no answers.

Ideomotor and Ideosensory Signals are fascinating and productive tools for bypassing the critical factor, the analytical mind that may otherwise intellectualize the responses, blocking the emergence of valid subconscious motives and knowledge.

It takes diligent practice to become proficient and comfortable with the use of these signals. It is well worth the effort to master these techniques. They will amaze the client and extract deeply hidden information that will be vital along the path to health and happiness.

CHAPTER 25

Inner Child Work

Inner Child work is that subcategory of Parts Therapy that deals with those aspects of the client that have been "stuck" in an earlier age. Due to traumatic events, resistance to maturing, or some other cause, the adult has fragments of their personality that subconsciously relate to the age they were when the events occurred.

The purpose of this technique is to assist these immature parts in their process of growing up or, in some cases, the resolution of emotions surrounding a trauma, thereby releasing any associated dysfunction.

Indications for Inner Child Work

The hypnotherapist will recognize the need for Inner Child work in various ways:

- When the client exhibits responses or language that are immature or inappropriate to their present age
- When the client refers to traumatic events in their past
- Following regression to cause
- When the client spontaneously regresses to an earlier age or event
- When the client states that their problem originated from an earlier incident in their life
- During a typical Parts Therapy session, when it is discovered that the dysfunctional or "misbehaving" part has an immature nature or is linked to an earlier age or event

Moving into Inner Child Work

When one of the above events occurs, ask the client how old they were during that event or how old they feel when behaving that way. If regression to cause has been accomplished, Inner Child work would begin at the age of the initial sensitizing event.

When they disclose the age, ask them to see that child or person they were at that time. If they describe a small child, ask them to imagine holding the child on their lap. If they were older, ask them to imagine sitting down comfortably together. When they say they have accomplished that, encourage or guide them through a dialogue with that younger person.

Though rare, there are clients who have shown disdain for the "child." They consider them an embarrassment or too painful to acknowledge. Occasionally, they bestow on that part of them the same abusive treatment that was experienced originally. This abandonment compounds the emotional distress of the "younger self." In some cases, release and healing can be produced simply by reconnecting the positive energy between the older and younger aspects, encouraging mutual support and nurturing.

Useful Questions

During the dialogue between the mature and the child parts, ask questions such as:

- What is it that this child needs at this time?
- What are they feeling?
- What can you do to help them feel better?
- Can you demonstrate to them that they will survive this situation?
- Can you let them see that you have grown up to be (safe, successful, loved, free, in control, etc.)?
- Can you acknowledge them and give them appreciation for the difficult times they went through in order for you to be here today?
- As hard as that time was, this young person was learning many valuable lessons that would add character and strength to your life. What was it that they learned by going through that event?
- What else do they need from you at this time?
- How are they feeling now?
- If they could give you their words of wisdom, what would they tell you?
- If you could share something special with them, what would it be?
- Is there anything else that you can do for them at this time?

Continue a similar line of questioning until the younger aspect of the client is fully satisfied and relieved. It may take some time. Allow your own creativity to discover ingenious perspectives from which to make this healing occur.

You will know the work is complete when the client reports such things as the younger self is happy, smiling, or relaxed or wants to take a nap or go out to play.

Maturing the Child

Alternatively, the client may agree that the child should mature to the present age. There are many ways to facilitate that perspective.

- Place the child part in one hand and the mature part in the other. Ask the client to bring those two parts together only so quickly as the child matures and reaches the full adult age. See chapter 28 for information on the Squash technique.
- Ask the client to imagine the child growing up and becoming the mature adult.
- Bring the child up through the different ages as the therapy proceeds, until all younger parts have arrived at the matured age.

It is not mandatory that the child part be matured to the present age. In some cases, the client will express the desire to allow them to remain at that age, now that the emotional dysfunctions attached to that age have been removed. The client may feel that the childlike aspect brings delight and wonder into their present experience. This determination is the prerogative of the client.

Bring the Healing into Other Ages

When the Inner Child issues at that age have been resolved, ask the client to go forward to the next time they could use some help. It is typical that these sessions touch on from one to a dozen distinct ages. The session may move through several stages of development from birth to the present age.

Although issues at each of these stages have been cleared, it can only be

> **Each presenting issue will have a string of specific correlating ages.**

assumed that these represent the ages that a particular issue surfaces. For instance, their challenges around low self-esteem have inner child links to ages two, five, eleven, twelve, eighteen, and thirty-six. When the client returns to your office to work on abandonment issues, they may regress to the crib, five, sixteen, twenty-two, and twenty-five.

Empowering the Child

It may be beneficial to have the client experience the Empowerment Symbol technique to discover a metaphorical gift that can be shared with the younger child. This can be very powerful in their bonding and in providing additional resources to the child to assist them through their tribulations. Refer to the chapters on Anchors and the Empowerment Symbol for complete descriptions of these techniques.

Facilitating Inner Child Work

1. Ask the client to remember at what age they first experienced the presenting issue or emotion.

2. Ask them to sit with the person they were at that age. Put the infant or toddler on their lap; older children and adults can sit together on the sofa or at a table.

3. The client will ask the younger aspect what they are feeling and will verbalize the response.

4. The client will ask the younger aspect what they need and will verbalize the response.

5. Discover the resolution to the crisis and provide it.

6. Acknowledge the wisdom and character traits the younger person acquired.

7. Facilitate the Empowerment Symbol, or other therapeutic techniques, if appropriate.

8. Continue until the younger aspect is completely satisfied.

9. Move to the next age when help is needed.

10. Continue until the present age.

Remember that the client chooses each of the ages that are addressed. Allow them to reveal what is needed and how they want the issue resolved. Sometimes a pillow is a useful prop for the client to hug while addressing the infant and small-child aspects.

We all have Inner Child work to do. The ages during which events occurred do not always have to be during childhood. A specific issue may have surfaced after the client began their career, or when their marriage failed.

Have a box of tissue handy. Inner Child work is powerful and typically results in the expression of many emotions.

Rare is the person who has arrived at adulthood unscathed by some event that has left an indelible imprint on that soul.

CHAPTER 26

Personality Part Retrieval

Personality Part Retrieval has many similarities to Inner Child work. Where Inner Child involves the altering of perspectives, or the releasing of memories and emotions surrounding events of an earlier age, Personality Part Retrieval requires regressing to an earlier age to recapture a trait or part of the personality or consciousness left behind. This condition is most likely due to trauma.

In this case, the client may complain of having lost their sense of innocence, trust, spontaneity, independence, joy, creativity, and so forth. In actuality, these traits are still present in the client. These parts of their personalities have simply been fragmented, hidden, blocked, forgotten, or discarded. The ritual of retrieving the trait gives the client permission to again exhibit it overtly. It is a beautiful and gratifying process to share with your client.

Retrieving the Part

As in Inner Child work, ask the client to return, in their imagination, to an earlier time when they still possessed that trait. When they have located that event, direct them to move forward in time, slowly, to when they notice that they no longer have that part.

Sometimes it is appropriate and advisable to have them move, in slow motion, across the threshold of that event several times, examining, at each passage, how the trait was left behind. Assist the client in learning whatever wisdom there is to be gained from that experience. This could involve the motives, perspectives, decision-making processes, etc., that were in effect at that time.

Request that the client create a metaphorical object that would represent this trait. Refer to the information about Object Imagery and submodalities given

Creating a metaphorical object that represents the recoverable trait allows the client to have a tangible object on which to focus.

earlier. This way, the trait becomes a tangible item that can be more readily manipulated. How do you find your innocence unless it has dimension? While this is a metaphorical consideration, it is also practical.

Reintegrating the Part

Once they have created the part's metaphorical appearance, the client can see it, touch it, hold it, and examine its qualities. Ask them to explore the possibilities that may occur should they decide to reintegrate this trait into their lives. How will their lives be different? What are the advantages and disadvantages of reintegration?

These possibilities are important to examine. The client may declare that they want their independence back but, when faced with it, may decide that they would likely leave their spouse and children. It is up to them to decide the effects their decisions will have on their lives and whether that is agreeable to them.

Some clients have decided that they would prefer to have the trait near them, accessible if the need arises, yet not fully integrated into their being at the present time. They are not ready for the consequences of reintegration.

For those who so choose, the next step involves the reintegration of the trait into their present conceptions of themselves. Ask them how they want to do that and where they want it "placed." This continues to keep the process completely client centered.

When they make the decision of how and where to place that part within them, give instructions to accomplish the reintegration. The client will know how to do it. When they inform you that it is done, ask them how they feel.

To properly conclude Personality Part Retrieval, facilitate Future Pacing with the client. This involves allowing them to envision going into the future with this newly recovered trait to imagine what future events will be like now that they have this resource. Future Pacing is more fully explained in chapter 28.

CHAPTER 27

Chair Therapy

Communication is one of the most important activities in which humans engage. It is also one of the most challenging aspects of relationships.

For many reasons, we withhold information, say too much, or incorrectly perceive other people's communications. All too often, we have been denied the opportunity to fully communicate our thoughts or bring closure to issues and relationships. These conditions can lead to frustration, anger, and sadness.

Chair Therapy can be a variation of Parts Therapy, particularly if the person in the other chair is an aspect of the client. However, more frequently the person in the other chair is another person with whom there is unsettled business.

When to Apply Chair Therapy

Chair Therapy will be appropriate in a number of situations. They include but are not limited to:

- When words have been left unsaid between the client and a person who is deceased.
- When the client is struggling with forgiveness for themselves or another person.
- When there are words that need to be said to another person, yet it would be inappropriate or inconvenient to speak to them directly.
- When the client would benefit from gaining another person's perspective.
- As an opportunity to gain wisdom from a perceived counselor or respected authority.

The benefits of Chair Therapy are plentiful. This technique gives the client the opportunity to release pent-up words or emotions, sort out internal conflict, and gain new perspectives and wisdom. The client can engage in this type of conversation with an unlimited range of people. When given the opportunity, clients have chosen to dialogue with co-workers, their boss, childhood bullies, abusers, experts in a field of study, a deceased friend or relative, or an alternative version of themselves.

This therapy technique works wonders when it is time to explore forgiveness. In allowing the client to express everything they have always wanted to say, there is relief, and closure can be experienced.

Setting Up Chair Therapy

When it becomes clear that the client is experiencing a block due to one of the above causes, Chair Therapy can be initiated either at the beginning of the session or, more likely, in the middle of it.

1. Determine with whom the client needs to speak—another person or themselves.

2. Ask the client to imagine that person sitting or standing before them.

3. Request that the client describe what they notice about that person. In doing so, the client begins to make a stronger connection with the process, clarifying their visualization of the person.

4. Inquire what the client would like to ask or tell the other person.

5. Ask the client to reveal the response they receive from the other person.

6. Continue in this manner until the client informs you that their issue is resolved.

7. Ask the client what they have learned from this experience and how they are feeling now.

8. Inquire if there is anything more to be resolved with this person, before moving on to another issue or closing the session.

9. On occasion, it is useful to have the client dissociate and move into the perspective of that other person. This allows them to gain the experience of someone who is observing them or has a different mindset.

When the client is satisfied with the resolution, proceed with other techniques or close the session.

Script for Calling on a Counselor

Occasionally, a client may need counsel from a person, living or dead, whom they deem to be extraordinarily wise. When this occurs, Chair Therapy is a handy tool to assist them in accomplishing their goal.

Clients have requested inspired answers from people such as Albert Einstein, Jesus, and Thomas Edison. The origins of the information they receive are indeterminate. Regardless, the responses are frequently inspired and useful.

In these cases, it is helpful to allow the client to describe a location where they would be comfortable speaking to the desired counselor. See chapter 11 for information on creating a safe space.

Once they have fully described the location and have gotten comfortable, introduce the counselor or guide to the client, and allow them to begin a dialogue. It may be helpful to know what questions the client is interested in having answered. This way, you can remind them of any that may be forgotten once the client is in trance.

The following is a script that could be used to guide your client to the point where they can begin the dialogue. After providing an induction of your choice, proceed as follows:

"I wonder if you can imagine a hallway stretching out before you. That hallway can look like anything that you want. And as you move down along that hallway, you begin to notice the texture of the floor covering beneath your feet. And the color of the walls. There are doorways along this hallway, each one leading to a special place. A place that will be most appropriate for you to encounter your preferred counselor. As I count from three to one, you will find yourself in front of one of these doors. Three, two, one.

"How would you describe the door where you are standing? (Pause for their description.)

"Are you ready to step through this door? (Client responds.) *Go ahead. Open the door and step through. Where do you find yourself? Outdoors or indoors?* (Pause for client response.) *Describe what you notice about your surroundings.* (Pause for client response.)

"Continuing to move through this scene, you find a comfortable place to sit down. You sit down there, going into a deep, deep meditation. It feels so good as you meditate. It is easy to become fully aware of your surroundings. Begin to notice your own energy and thoughts. Observing. Aware and connected.

"As you continue sitting there, you notice that your counselor begins to move towards you. Feel them moving closer. You can sense your counselor as they sit down beside you. Perhaps you can see them now. Observe their appearance, whether through vision or sensing. If they have hair, what would it be like? What would be the color of their eyes? Observe their clothing and anything unusual about them. You are fully present there, with this wise person. Begin to have a conversation with your counselor now. Feel free to verbalize your thoughts and words, as you ask your questions and receive their response."

Continue to guide them through their conversation, assisting them with any of the questions that they may forget to ask. When the conversation is complete and the client has no more questions, ask them to thank their counselor for being available to them today and for kindly answering the questions. Then you may close the session.

Chair Therapy is helpful in resolving issues that involve third parties who are absent from the session. It assists the client in putting closure on past relationships, resolving forgiveness issues, and gaining the perspective or wisdom of another person.

CHAPTER 28

Outcome-Based Therapies

There are a number of therapies that require the client to extrapolate a reasonable procession of events, or outcomes, should they continue on a given path. These techniques assist in the discovery of what lies beyond immediate gratification, fear, or habit. They allow the client to understand and take responsibility for their decisions and actions.

What Is at the Core?

Core states are conditions that we, as humans, strive for in our lives. We actually have access to these core states any time, as they are a part of our essential being. Our experience of these core states becomes clouded, blocked, forgotten, ignored, or denied through our perceptions of, and reactions to, life's events. With this technique, we are able to identify that core state, access it, and bring it back into our daily experiences.

Core states are those that have no further goal or purpose. They represent the final goal. These many include:

- Love
- Peace
- Being
- Oneness
- Wholeness
- Happiness
- Pure Consciousness

A word of caution: The core state of Love is not the same as being in love. The core state of Being has nothing to do with

> **Core states are permanent, all-encompassing states that are a final and ultimate goal.**

doing. Happiness, in this context, is not the same as being happy, which may be transitory.

Who Will Benefit from Accessing a Core State?

Any client will benefit who complains of behaviors that they wish to alter or be rid of.

- Addictions—Smoking, food, alcohol, drugs, shopping, sex, etc.
- Other compulsive behaviors—Hypervigilance, overanalyzing, kleptomania
- Emotional responses—Anger, rage, defensiveness, violence, cowering
- Blocks to success—In business, finances, personal relationships, spiritual issues
- Health issues—Chronic pain, symptoms, or conditions
- Life choices—Poor decisions, indecision

Outcome-based techniques benefit anyone addressing issues in their life. These techniques can even be self-administered, by asking yourself the prescribed series of questions and writing down your responses.

Revelations at the Core

Assisting a client in accessing their core state is a process that can be administered on its own or combined with other techniques, to gain rapid progress in the healing process and enhance the effectiveness of the session.

The technique is used to gain access to the true core state that the person, or part of them, is striving to achieve. This core state is frequently hidden behind clumsy or dysfunctional behaviors that are distasteful to the client.

When a part of the client is acting out in a way that makes them uncomfortable—whether in behavior, physical health, or emotions—this simple technique will help them understand their response and begin the process of changing towards a more desirable response.

A Part Is Revealed

When a client complains of a behavior that they want to change, the vigilant hypnotherapist will automatically detect a parts issue. There is a part of them that displays the said behavior and another part of them that has brought them into your office to change it.

Although not necessary, there is a benefit in setting this up as Parts Therapy. Following the formula described in the chapter on Parts Therapy, the part that displays this behavior would be separated out and placed on one of the client's hands. This makes it easier for that part to respond to the questions more purely. The part that creates the disturbing behavior is the one to address.

Accessing the Core State

In the script example that follows, there is a client, Dan, who wants to quit smoking. Change the words accordingly for alternative issues that your respective clients present. Begin by asking the following:

"Is it true for you that there is a part of you that would like to quit smoking and another part of you that resists that effort? (Client responds positively.) *I wonder if you can imagine separating those two parts so that the part of you that wishes to quit smoking is on one of your hands . . . and the part that resists that effort is on the other hand. Please indicate to me when you have accomplished that.* (Client responds positively.) *And please indicate which hand has the part that wants to quit smoking.* (Client responds, "Right.") *And the left hand has the part that is resisting?"* (Client responds affirmatively.)

Once the part has been separated and can be addressed directly, the next step is to give it assurances, respect, and support. Explain that you and the client understand that its intentions are positive. You know that it feels it is doing the best it can for the good of the whole person, who is the client. The objective is to win its confidence, not to alienate it or push it into a defensive stance.

If it is truly a part of the client, then the ultimate goal of that part will be aligned with what it feels is the highest good of the client. Its methods of achieving it are simply proving to be less than fruitful. Thus, you are both on the same team; there are simply some tactical issues to resolve. Continue:

"I would like to assure the part in the left hand, the part that has resisted all efforts Dan has attempted in quitting smoking, that we understand that it is doing the best it can. We understand that its intentions are good, and that it has been striving to achieve something for Dan that it deems to be positive and supportive of Dan's life. Dan, by understanding more fully the motivations the left hand has in wanting to continue to smoke, we will be able to discover how we can work together to successfully attain those goals for the benefit of the whole body. I would like you to now go into the left hand. Imagine that you are fully this part, with all its emotions, feelings, thoughts, motivations, and desires. And when you have done so, please describe to me what you are experiencing."

The Intended Goal

The next step is to discover the part's intended goal.

"Please explain to me: In encouraging Dan to continue smoking, what goal do you want to achieve for him?"

Listen to its response. Record this response in your notes.

Next, we will determine the rest of the Outcome chain, by repeatedly asking the following question:

"If you were to attain _____ [the above goal], fully, just the way that you want it, then what would you want that is even more important?"

Record the client's response.

Repeat this line of questioning, recording each answer in order, until you reach the core state. When they respond with a word from the above list of core states, or if they say that there is nothing further they would want, you have reached their ultimate goal for this behavior.

Anchoring the Core State

When the core state has been discovered, direct the client to fully experience the sensations of achieving their goal. Most likely, they have not attained this sensation from any of the dysfunctional behavioral methods they were previously using.

At this point, it is productive to anchor this feeling in whatever manner you prefer. You may discover that the

> **The experience of this ultimate goal is generally very exhilarating for the client.**

Empowerment Symbol is an elegant way to achieve this.

"As you are experiencing this core state right now, I wonder if you can truly feel it at all levels of your being. Connect with this state, enhancing it fully . . . turning up the volume . . . that's right. And as you are experiencing it right now, fully, I wonder if your subconscious mind will present to you a symbol that would represent this feeling. A symbol you could perhaps imagine holding in your hand. (Pause.) *And what do you notice?"*

The client will respond with a symbol such as a sun, star, waterfall, beam of light, medallion, etc.

"This state of being, this sense of _____ [core state], is already a part of you. You have already attained it and it is yours forever. You can walk in this state of _____ each and every day in everything that you experience. And anytime you feel that you need assistance in accessing this state of _____, you can easily recall it by simply imagining this symbol that you hold in your hand right now."

Reversing the Outcome Chain

Once the core state has been achieved, bring that state of being into each of the Outcomes, in reverse order. This allows the client to discover a new way of perceiving and experiencing the various intermediary goals that it previously desired. This is where the real transformation begins.

"You may now carry this symbol and this sensation of _____ [core state] with you into each and every experience that you have. And as you experience this _____ now, and carry this _____ [symbol] with you, how does that change your experience of _____ [the last item on your Outcome chain list]?"

Direct the client to bring that core state with them, along with the symbol of that state, into the experience of each Outcome along the chain.

Begin with that last one and work your way up to the original goal of the undesirable behavior or response.

"And now, bringing that sensation of _____ [core state] with you, along with your _____ [symbol], how does that change your experience of the need to continue smoking?"

Typically, the client will express an overwhelming acknowledgment that there is no need for that original behavior whatsoever. Transformation has been accomplished!

Conclude the Process

Once the part that has created the dysfunctional behavior has agreed that its present modality no longer is productive or necessary, it is probably willing to

> **Clients frequently describe their sensations of this transformation, using words such as "great," "relieved," "energized," and "excited."**

fully cooperate with the rest of the client that sought the change. Follow the procedures delineated in Parts Therapy for reintegration of the parts.

The Squash

Now that the client has discovered they already had this state of being, this desired core state, within them all along, they will be pleased to be able to share this perspective with all their past and future experiences. The Squash achieves rapid integration.

"I wonder if you can imagine holding your symbol in your right hand, while experiencing this sense of _____ [core state]. This right hand represents you, now, at your present age, experiencing this new learning. Now, imagine that your left hand contains your earliest childhood memories. Do you sense that now? I would like you to bring these two hands together only so quickly as this state of _____ moves through all of your life experiences, through all the years and events. Allow all the awareness and learning of that sense of _____ to integrate and become a part of each and every experience, every memory, and every event throughout your entire life. That's right, just bringing your hands together, as this

state of _____ becomes an integral part of each moment. All the feelings, perceptions, awareness, are filtering, now, through this sense of _____. Integrating and bringing these experiences together, in their natural state. That's right. Fully integrated, feeling so good."

As the client collapses their newly integrated learning into all of their life experiences, they will typically experience a wonderful shift in their perceptions of their childhood and their earlier adult life. They may experience a shift in how they have perceived events and other people in their life, as well as how they view themselves.

Alternatively, the core state and Empowerment Symbol could be carried into past events through Inner Child techniques. The client carries these newly retrieved traits into pivotal past events, sharing them with the younger version of themselves.

Follow the reorientation of the past with questions that will allow you to learn how they anticipate handling future events, now that they have transformed old behaviors. This is an important step. The client has decided that they no longer want the dysfunctional behavior, and steps have been taken to accomplish this. Their perceptions of the past have been altered with this knowledge. Now, through Future Pacing, we will facilitate their sense of comfort in handling future circumstances.

Sample of Future Pacing for the Core State

"I wonder if you can imagine moving ahead in time. In a short while, you will be leaving this office and going to your next destination. Describe to me what you anticipate will be different about that experience now that you have your symbol and your renewed sense of _____ [core state]."

Allow the client to describe how they foresee that future event.

"Now, allow yourself to imagine moving out into the future about a week. What do you notice about yourself in a week from now?"

Repeat this same line of questioning, using various future time intervals, such as three months, six months, one year, five years. This allows the client to imagine a new and more positive future, which in turn more easily allows it to become reality.

Summary of Accessing the Core State

This therapy technique is effectively used entirely on its own or in combination with other techniques such as Parts Therapy, Inner Child work, and Regression therapy. You may find it to be one of the more effective tools you have at your disposal. Following are the steps for setting up the therapy.

- Determine the behavior or condition the client wants transformed.
- Isolate that behavior or condition as a "part."
- Show respect and support for the part, assuming that it is doing the best it can.
- Ask the part what it wants for the client, its goal.
- Ask the part, if it were to achieve that goal, fully, what would it then have, or want, which is even more important.
- Continue that line of questioning, writing down each response in order, until the part reaches a core state of being—Love, Peace, Being, Oneness, Wholeness, Happiness, Pure Consciousness, for example.
- Amplify the experience of that core state of being.
- Ask the subconscious mind to create a symbol that would represent that state of being.
- Request that the client carry that symbol and that core state of being with them into the experience of the previous Outcome states, starting at the last one and moving up the list in reverse order.
- Ask them to carry that symbol and that core state of being with them into the experience of the undesired behavior or condition.
- Integrate the part with the whole of the client.
- Collapse this new learning into the experience and perceptions of the past.
- Future Pace, carrying this symbol and new learning into anticipated future events.

This may appear to be a lengthy process. Once it has become mastered, it moves quickly and achieves a rapid shift in the person's state of being.

Other Outcome-Based Therapies

Many approaches will achieve results similar to the core states technique. They are variations of what can be termed Outcome chains.

An Outcome chain would involve choosing a behavior or a desired goal and asking the client, *"If you were to achieve that goal, what outcome do you hope to gain?"* When the client responds, ask this question again. Continue to ask the question after each response until a final outcome is obtained.

The Outcome chain is a helpful therapy when a client is trying to understand the results of their behaviors and decisions. By proceeding through the Outcome chain, the client has the opportunity to look ahead into the future and take responsibility for the consequences of their actions and choices.

What If?

Other techniques that can achieve a similar result are less structured. They use variations of the phrase, *"What if?"* They can be used in response to distorted perceptions and generalizations that the client may present.

For example, when a client says, "I can't do that" or "I'll never do that," respond by asking, *"What would happen if you did?"* With each client response, counter with another question: *"And then what would happen?"* Frequently, the client is able to realize that the benefits of doing what they deemed impossible or not acceptable to others may outweigh the disappointment over not attempting it.

The Worst-Case Scenario

A "belief buster" can be delivered when clients artificially limit themselves based on fear. Ask the question, *"What is the worst thing that could happen if you were to [move ahead, go through that door, speak your mind, do something just for you, etc.]?"* When they respond, counter with, *"What would be the worst thing that could happen if that happened?"* Continue with that line of inquiry until the client realizes that, typically, the worst they can imagine happening would have little or no real consequence in their life.

> **Fears are rarely a reflection of reality.**

CHAPTER 29

Reframing

Occasionally, when working with parts, the client will agree that the part that is causing the unwanted behavior is willing to change. However, it is unable to determine what choices are available or how to implement a change. It feels that it has always done things one way, or reacted to situations in a consistent manner, and now realizes that the chosen course of action is not achieving the desired results. Yet that part has difficulty seeing beyond its own limitations to discover an alternative, and more fruitful, course of action.

Reframing presents the client with the opportunity to expand on their creativity and resources, to ascertain a list of possibilities from which to now choose.

Reframing will be helpful in the following cases:

- When the client feels that there are no choices available to them to change unwanted behaviors
- Anytime the client wants to cross the boundaries of their own limitations in order to find creative solutions and generate fresh ideas

Reframing is easily executed during Parts Therapy or as an exercise on its own.

Steps for Reframing

1. The client discloses the nature of the problem or unwanted behavior.
2. Separate the problem, or behavior, from the positive purpose that it serves.
3. Ask the client to generate new solutions or alternatives.

4. Evaluate the solutions.

5. Choose one solution to implement that is practical, achieves the desired objective, and is readily available to the client.

6. Reinforce with Future Pacing and other techniques.

The Creative Link

Finding alternative solutions to life's dilemmas requires creativity. It is possible that an individual has cloaked their creativity because of inhibitions, fear of failing, or fear of being mocked. Others are avoiding the weight of responsibility and practicality. Creativity is a chaotic and compelling force.

When delivering this therapy, allow your voice to become dramatic and persuasive. Hearing the emotion in your voice, the client will begin to give themselves permission to be expressive and artistic as well. This will enhance their openness to new experiences and allow the flow of ideas.

Sample Script for Reframing

When the client has disclosed the nature of the unwanted behavior, lead them through an induction and deepening, and then proceed:

"I would like to speak to the part of you that controls this behavior . . . that part that chooses to _____ [name behavior]. We understand that this part has done everything it can to provide a benefit to _____ [client's name].

"In speaking with that part that has created this behavior, I would like to ask you to reveal to the conscious mind the benefits, the positive function, that you hope to gain for _____ [client's name]. (Wait for client's response.)

"We realize that the function you are serving has a benefit, a positive function that is beneficial to _____ [client's name]. Your goal is positive, yet there may be a way that this goal could be achieved that is even more effective and beneficial. Would you be willing to explore these possibilities if you know that you are, in no way, obligated to accept or choose an alternative behavior?" (Pause for client's response.)

Recruit the Creative Part

"I wonder if you would agree that there is another part of you that is very creative. (Pause for confirmation.) *I would like to ask that creative*

part of you to fully experience the energy and essence of that creativity, now.

"Perhaps you remember the wonder and amazement you experienced as a child, when your imagination runs wild with ideas, make-believe, stories, and dreams. It was so fun to just play and daydream, to fantasize about life, your future, and who you are. Perhaps you remember drawing and painting, creating images, choosing colors.

"And perhaps your creative nature remembers playing make-believe, when the roles you play come alive. You really were the cowboy, the warrior, the king of the mountain [or the princess, the teacher, the mommy]. Perhaps you even imagined yourself to be an animal, and you really felt like that lion, or that monkey, or that horse. And while you were that animal, you moved like that animal. You could even make sounds like that animal. And your imagination makes it all so real.

"Do you ever wonder if you can remember when you have created art, or written a poem, or listened to music? A time when you generated new ideas, new ways of expressing yourself. And something inside of you feels so exhilarated and focused. Notice how you feel as you remember those events, now.

"That's right. You are creative, and it feels so good, and so right, to connect with that part of you. Energizing that creativity, experiencing that wonder and amazement, the expansion of thoughts and ideas. That's right. It feels so good, so natural."

Warping Time

"I know that you have, at one time or another, in your life, experienced the feeling that time is not a constant. Sometimes it seems as though time moves very quickly, and at other times, time moves so slow. And it is true; the movement of time is a part of our imagination. And there is a part of your subconscious mind that knows this, even if consciously it is hard to understand.

"I would like to ask that part of your mind that understands this to travel through time and space, taking the creative aspect of your mind with it. It can take all the time it needs, and travel to the ends of the universe if it wants, in order to bring back to you a list of at least ten ideas—solutions—that you can consider as choices in the issue we have been discussing. The solutions and choices your subconscious mind brings to you may be unusual, impractical, silly, or fantastical. Or they may be

viable, imaginative, and ingenious! It really does not matter. They are simply ideas, choices, creative solutions that will allow you to consider alternative pathways. A new course of action and possibilities for your future.

"I would like to ask the subconscious part that knows how to travel through time and space, along with the creative part, to take all the time that it needs, going wherever it wants and yet to return here, with these new ideas in the space of time that it takes me to count from three to one. Going there now. (Pause for about five seconds and then count slowly.) *Three . . . two . . . one."*

Revealing the Possibilities

"I would now like to ask those parts of your subconscious mind that have retrieved the list of solutions to now reveal, to the conscious mind, what it has discovered. Go ahead and tell _____ [client's name] what you now know about the items on the list. (Pause for response.)

"What other ideas can you think of? (Pause for response.)

"You may find it fascinating to evaluate each of the choices you have listed. Of those solutions, which ones are immediately available to you, and as effective as your present behavior? (Pause for response.)

"Of the available and effective solutions, which one would you consider the most satisfying? (Pause for response.)

"I would like to ask the part that has previously been producing the unwanted behavior if it would be willing to try that. (Pause for response.)

"In what way can you imagine implementing that course of action?" (Pause for response.)

Future Pacing

"Now, take this new behavior, and move ahead in time, into the future. Go into the future where you have already fully incorporated this new behavior, fully in the context of your environment and lifestyle. What do you notice about that imaginary future scene? (Pause for response.)

"Is this new response or behavior a satisfactory solution? Will it be immediately available and effective in the situations that previously caused the unwanted behavior? (If yes, move to the next step. If no, go back and choose another solution, or continue to generate new viable choices.)

"*Please go inside and discover whether there is a part of you that would be willing to be responsible for the implementation of this new choice.* (Pause for response.)

"*Anytime in the future, should this new behavior no longer serve its function, or should the old behavior reappear, it will be a natural reminder that it is time for the subconscious mind to simply generate a new and more useful solution.*"

Continuing with Other Techniques

From this point, proceed with other techniques to reinforce this new learning. These may involve:

- Role Model—To learn how someone else, or a future aspect of the client, achieved this solution.
- Desensitization—To dispel any fear around this course of action.
- Parts Therapy—To discover any part that would sabotage this new decision.
- Empowerment Symbol or Anchoring—To install beneficial resources that will support their choice.
- Swish—To reinforce the new behavioral reactions.

Creating New Responses

Reframing a problematic behavior is a means of generating alternative behaviors and choices that will obtain the same objective, without the destructive side effects of the old behavior. Similar to Outcome-based techniques, it targets the purpose, not the behavior itself. Reframing offers one step further to discover and incorporate new behavioral responses.

CHAPTER 30

Dissociation

"Associated" and "dissociated" are terms that refer to the point of reference or perspective held by the client. Associated indicates that they are
in the first person, looking out through "their eyes" while reliving the
experience. Dissociated means that the client is viewing the experience as
an observer, a third party, from a perspective outside of their own body.

While dissociation occurs naturally as a normal part of the human
experience, there are times when it is advantageous to activate dissociation as a part of the healing process. Dissociation may be indicated when
the event to be examined is too charged with negative emotion for the
client to experience while in the associated state.

> **The purpose for applying dissociation is to achieve distance
> from the experience of a traumatic even while reviewing it,
> or to understand another peson's position and perspective.**

When to Apply Dissociation

A client may achieve dissociation spontaneously while in regression.
This is their subconscious means of protecting themselves. Alternatively,
dissociation can be facilitated when warranted.

Dissociation is advised in cases of:

• Trauma
• Phobia

When it is advisable to assist the client into the dissociated state, it can
be achieved in a number of ways:

- Ask the client to view the event as though they were watching from a corner of the room.
- Use the theatrical device described below.
- It may be appropriate for them to take the perspective of another person, by "stepping into their body." This would be helpful when there is a need for the client to understand how others see them, or when another person's perspective will aid in resolution of a problem.

> **A client complained that because she was petite, everyone treated her as a child. During the therapy, she was asked to slip out of her own body and into the body of her co-worker, who was tall. By doing so, the client was able to see how different it felt to be tall, even discovering for herself that she would feel strange and awkward at that height. She further felt that the co-worker was not really treating her as a child. She discovered that her own "colored glasses," which filtered her perceptions, were tainting her experiences at work.**

The Theater Method of Dissociation

The following is an example of a visualization technique that may be used or improvised to achieve dissociation for the client. This is particularly helpful in addressing cataclysmic, traumatic, and phobic issues.

"Allow your eyes to gently drift closed. Breathing . . . and relaxing . . . that's right.

"I wonder if you can imagine walking into a movie theater. It can look like anything that you wish. As you walk into that theater, you notice the rows and rows of empty seats. Allow yourself to find a seat near the middle of the theater. Sit down in one of the chairs and get comfortable.

"That's right . . . feeling so good. Relaxed and comfortable.

"Now, I wonder if you can imagine yourself just lifting up off your body . . . that's right . . . floating right up out of your body. Drift back and up into the projection room. That's right, allow yourself to simply float up, and into the projection room.

"From this perspective, you are able to look out the little window, down into the audience, and discover your body sitting there, in that middle row, looking towards the screen. That's right. Notice the back of

your head as you see yourself sitting there in that seat.

"Here you are, in the projection room, noticing the back of your head, as your body watches the screen. That's right. Very good.

"As you continue to watch the back of your head, you notice out of the corner of your eye that the curtain is opening and the movie is about to begin. As the film begins to roll, you notice that it is a movie about that event in the past that we have been discussing. Just continue to watch the back of your head, as that body in the middle row watches the film. Very good.

"Allow the film to run all the way past the end of that event, to when you realize that you are safe. Tell me when it has done so. Very good. Now continue watching the back of your head, as the film is run backwards, through the entire episode, until it is back at the beginning of the event. Back at the beginning, when you were feeling good, before the event occurred.

"Very good. Now allow the film to run forward again, all the way through the episode . . . until the event is complete and you know that you have survived it and are OK.

"Very good. Now let the film run backwards again, all the way to the beginning, to before the event began. That's right."

Wait for a Shift

Watch the client closely. If they are showing signs that they are still traumatized by this event, repeat these steps at least once more while they view it from the projection room. When they appear to be relaxing, becoming more comfortable with this event, proceed.

"I wonder if you can now imagine yourself floating back out of the projection room, right back down and into your body, sitting there in the middle row of the theater. That's right, just floating back down . . . down . . . into your body, feeling the chair there in the middle row, and looking up at the screen. Very good.

"Once again, the projector starts the film, moving through the event, watching the movie. That's right. Just continue to watch the film as it rolls through the event. Until it is over and you know that you are safe again. Very good. How are you feeling?

"Allow the film to move backwards through the episode once again. That's right. Going backwards through the event, all the way to the beginning, to before the event began. Very good.

"The film starts again, and this time, as you watch the film, what do you notice that is different? What are you beginning to observe about this event?"

The questions are designed to elicit insights, wisdom, new learning, and resources that are beginning to become apparent to the client. Frequently, they are verbalizing the event forward, then rewinding, and verbalizing forward again a number of times. This serves an additional purpose of desensitizing them while they are in the dissociated state.

"Very good. You are back at the beginning again, when you were feeling good. To before the event began. That's right.

"I wonder if you can now imagine standing up in the theater and walking to the screen. Walking right up to the front of the theater, and stepping right into the screen, into that movie, into the you that is moving through that event.

"Very good. How are you feeling? All right. Now, this time I want you to move through that episode from the perspective of being in your own body, looking out through your own eyes. That's right. Very good. What are you noticing now about that event?

"Moving backwards through the event, until you reach the beginning, how do you feel now? OK. Moving once again through the event, all the way to the end. That's right. Moving through. Very good. How do you feel now?"

Points for Successful Dissociation

- Notice that the client went through each stage two times. That is the minimum required. Be sensitive in determining how many more times may be needed.
- Frequently inquire how the client is feeling. Remember that the whole exercise may involve them describing their experiences, which can be an intellectual exercise. Encourage them to connect with their emotions also.
- Pay attention to the ways in which the story begins to change after a few narrations.
- Notice that this script creates two stages of dissociation for the client. One is the perspective from the projection room, and the other is from the theater seat. This creates a very safe space for the client to work

through the details of a traumatic event. Barriers have been created to protect them personally from the fear that surrounds that issue.
• Many variations may be added to this visualization, utilizing additional tools and resources to create deep and lasting change.
—Allow the client to take an Empowerment Symbol with them.
—Dress the antagonist of the story in comical clothing.
—Give the client superpowers.
—Turn the "villain" into a cartoon character.
—Suggest they take a friend or a hero with them.
—Make up a better, more positive, story to replace this one.

Setting Up the Theater Method of Dissociation

1. Create a visualization of a theater.
2. The client visualizes entering and sitting in a center row.
3. The client imagines floating up, out of their body, and into the projection room (dissociates).
4. They watch the back of their head, as the body watches the screen.
5. The movie of the traumatic event begins.
6. Move forward and backwards at least twice, while the client is watching the back of the head.
7. The client imagines floating back into the body in the center of the theater and views the event like a movie.
8. Move through the story forward and backwards at least twice again.
9. The client imagines walking up to the screen and stepping into the event (associates).
10. Move forward and backwards through the episode at least twice again.

The client is ready to be re-associated whenever they are prepared to experience the event from the first-person perspective. Do not attempt to do it prematurely. Continue the dissociated processes until they confirm that they are relaxed and comfortable enough with the situation to proceed to the associated state.

CHAPTER 31

Desensitization

Desensitization is another technique used for treatment of trauma, phobia, and any highly charged event that elicits emotions such as rage, anger, grief, etc. The purpose is to lower the impact that the event or situation has on the client, thereby restoring balance in their responses.

We have all been told, "You will get over it in time." Frequently, during high-impact events, the newness or shock of the situation magnifies its intensity. Once the person becomes accustomed to the idea of it, it "wears off," lowering the impact.

To facilitate desensitization, simply instruct the client to recount the episode repeatedly, creating a sense of boredom in

> **People naturally practice desensitization when they repeat emotionally charged stories of their lives over and over again.**

the client. After a while, the story loses its intensity and another story replaces it.

Desensitization, as a therapy method, allows the emotional charge to dissipate rapidly, removing the need for time to pass. All the time needed will occur in the course of the session.

Accomplishing Desensitization

This is accomplished by instructing the client to describe the situation in detail, from beginning to end. When they have completed their story, have them repeat it again, in detail. Continue requesting the repetition of the story until they indicate that they are bored or getting aggravated at the exercise. Then have them do it one more time.

By the end, you should be detecting boredom, apathy, or resignation in their voice. Gone are the highly charged expletives, the emotional outbursts, discomfort, and negativity.

Throughout the session, keep your line of questions client centered and nonleading. The sequence of the questions will be similar to the following:

1. Tell me what happened to make you so upset.
2. What happened next?
3. Did anything else happen?
4. Run the story backwards in your mind to just before the beginning again.
5. Tell me the story again.
6. What happened next?
7. Do you notice anything else about that story?
8. Run the story backwards to the beginning again.
9. This time, tell me the story as though you were moving through it in slow motion.
10. What do you notice this time?
11. What are your feelings as you move through the story this time?
12. Run the story backwards again to the beginning.
13. As you tell me the story this time, what do you notice that is different or unexpected?
14. How do you feel now?
15. Run the story backwards again to the beginning.
16. Tell me the story again, adding any details that you may have left out previously.
17. What do you notice about the story this time?
18. Run the story backwards again to the beginning.

It is obvious where this line of questioning is going. Depending on the situation or the events that have taken place, you may find that certain other questions or tactics will be useful.

These may include questions concerning what the client learned, what wisdom they gained from the experience, what responsibility they need to accept, or what responsibility is not theirs to carry.

During desensitization, it may be useful to add devices suggested in the Theater Method of Dissociation—humorous visualizations, a fresh perspective, anchors to positive resources, and so forth.

This technique is suitable for many issues—from a teenager upset over losing her first love to soldiers coming home from battle with posttraumatic stress disorder. The hardest part is requiring the client to tell the story one last time—after they have expressed how tedious the exercise has become. That is when you truly know you have accomplished your mission!

CHAPTER 32

The Swish

The Swish is a versatile tool that has taken many individualized forms. No matter how it is set up, what visual scene is set to accomplish it, the Swish is effective in creating rapid behavioral modification.

The purpose of the Swish is to create new and resourceful, healthier and wiser responses in your client. It is the tool of choice for generating new behaviors.

> **If your client says that every time she starts her car, she lights up a cigarette, yet she would prefer to drink water, the Swish is the natural tool to use.**

In every case, the groundwork needs to be laid first. The Swish is very effective with weight-loss and smoking clients, but only after they have been regressed to root cause, have eliminated all the secondary gains, and have had conversations with their "parts" to assure they are all on the winning side. When the only thing left to do is to remove automatic behaviors, it is time to bring in the Swish!

Facilitating the Swish

A trance state is not required to facilitate this technique. If the client is already under hypnosis, you are ready to go. If not, just have them close their eyes.

This script would be appropriate for someone who wants to drink water instead of smoke a cigarette when driving a car. Change the images appropriately to suit the goals of your client.

Three key questions need to be answered before you begin:

• When do you exhibit the negative behavior? *When driving.*
• What triggers your behavior? *Turning the key in the ignition.*
• What would you prefer to do? *Drink water.*

The Steps

1. Find out the response the client wishes to remove.
2. Discover under what circumstances it is exhibited.
3. Learn the exact trigger for the response.
4. Determine what response the client prefers.
5. Ask them to close their eyes and relax.
6. Request that they imagine two pictures—one shows the moment of receiving the trigger that elicits the response to be removed, and the other exhibits the desired response.
7. Instruct the client to imagine one picture in each of their hands, and to disclose which hand has which picture.
8. Guide the client through the visualization described in the script below, repeating the last paragraph a minimum of eight to ten times.
9. Ask them how they feel.
10. Break state—talk about a different subject for a minute or two.
11. Make an environmental check
12. Have the client emerge from trance.

Sample Script for the Swish

"Closing your eyes, and relaxing. I wonder if you can imagine holding two pictures. One picture will be of that moment as you put the key in the ignition of your car. The other picture will be of you grabbing your bottle of water and taking a drink. Can you see those two pictures? Which hand has the picture of you starting your car? (Right hand.) *OK. And the picture of you taking the water and drinking is in your left hand.* (Yes.) *Very good.*

"I want you to look at the picture in your right hand. As you look at it, you notice that it begins to turn yellow. It fades like an old picture. Shrinking down, ever smaller, until it becomes a dot and disappears. Do you see that? (Nod.) *Very good.*

"Now, look at the picture in your left hand. As you look at it, allow it

to become brighter, more colorful and vivid, as it grows larger and larg-
er. So large that you can step right into the picture, as you pick up that
bottle of water and take a drink. So refreshing, wet and cool. That's right,
feeling so good to be doing something so good just for you. Can you feel
that? (Nod) *Very good.*

"*We will be doing this exercise again, each time faster and faster*
because your subconscious learns at a very rapid pace. Here we go.

"*Take a look at the picture in your right hand. See it fade, shrink, and dis-*
appear, as you look at the picture in your left hand. It becomes so colorful,
vivid, growing larger and larger, so large that you step in, and take a sip of
water. Feeling so good. Take a deep breath in . . . hold it . . . and release."

Repeat the above paragraph at least eight to ten times. It can be done
even more times if necessary. The only way to determine the number of
repetitions necessary is to be intuitive and sensitive. The purpose of the
repetitions is to bind the subconscious mind to a new habit that replaces
an old one.

Breaking State

When you have com-
pleted enough repetitions,
break state. This lets the
client get their mind off
the exercise and their
desired goals.

> **Breaking state means that you change
> the subject and engage in an unrelated
> conversation for about a minute.**

After a minute or so of conversation, perform an environmental check
by asking them to tell you a story about what they imagine will happen
the next time they are in a previously triggering situation. You may state,
"*We are about at the end of our session. In a few moments, you will be
leaving this office. Tell me what you imagine will happen when you get
into your car.*"

Chances are the goals
have been achieved if
they say that they will
start their car and take a
drink of water as they
drive away. If they

> **An environmental check allows the
> hypnotherapist to determine whether
> the changes will hold when the client
> experiences a triggering event.**

respond that they will be fighting the urge to have a cigarette, it will be obvious that the work is not yet complete. Perhaps there is a need to continue with the Swish a few more times, or address secondary gains that have not yet been eliminated.

Summary of the Swish

The Swish is a rapid method for creating new behavioral responses to stimuli. It can be used in cases involving habits, such as procrastination, overeating, and smoking. It is also effective in altering emotional responses such as anger, aggression, and inhibition. This technique attempts to break old habits and create new pathways to more desirable responses.

Practice the Swish sufficiently so that you can do it without reading the script. If you are picturing the whole process in your mind, clearly, you will be intimate with the procedure and fully engaged with the client's experience.

CHAPTER 33

Anchors

At birth, each human being exhibits great strength of will. We are all uninhibited. Have you ever seen a baby being shy about signaling their mother to satisfy their immediate needs? Have you witnessed a baby being embarrassed about needing their diaper changed?

Somewhere along the way, our inherent sense of self-care and the will to achieve our fundamental purpose become diluted or convoluted or simply vanish. That innate knowledge and force is tainted by our experiences and perception of life.

Where does it go? What happened to it? Is it irretrievable?

> **If the trait can be imagined, it already resides at some level within the person.**

The good news is that these traits can be recovered. It is possible to reclaim aspects of ourselves that we have left behind. We can even capture qualities that we have never exhibited—characteristics that we have only seen in other people.

How can this be accomplished? Using anchors, we can regain, or create, powerful forces within each one of us.

Risking Change

Whenever higher standards are set for oneself, stepping out of the comfort zone is required. A person has to be willing to strive, work, and do what it takes to accomplish the desired goal.

Change becomes most threatening to people who find themselves comfortable. Typically, when a person is comfortable, they do everything they can to maintain status quo. They defend and protect their position, and this may result in maintaining an undesirable path. This, in turn, increases fear of change and the unknown. The character weakens, self-esteem diminishes, and doubt sets in. It becomes harder and harder to make a change. Yet, change is required for advancement.

In fact, change is our friend! Change brings better things—growth, increased wealth, a raise or promotion, and so forth. Without change, our dreams cannot become reality. Yet, there is the risk of loss, embarrassment, or being wrong. It is a risk that has to be managed, and a risk that eventually has to be taken.

So when your client is ready, or sees the need, to make a change, anchoring positive strengths and resources will allow them

> **Imagine what changes you will experience as you become a successful hypnotherapist.**

to proceed with greater confidence and enthusiasm.

What Is an Anchor?

An anchor is anything that connects the conscious awareness to something else, most likely a memory of an event, a person, or a feeling. Our lives are filled with anchors.

For example, what happens to you when you:

• Smell bread baking?
• Look at photos of a vacation?
• Hear the name of someone who caused you great pain?
• Taste a food you only eat during special holidays?

We are inundated with anchors everyday. Some of them produce positive, happy responses; some of them conjure negative

> **Anchors elicit memories and arouse emotions that correlate to events from the past.**

thoughts, behaviors, and feelings. Through techniques of hypnotherapy, we are able to collapse or neutralize the negative anchors, and create or enhance positive ones. We will be discussing how that works in just a moment.

What Creates an Anchor?

Any stimulus of a sensory pathway that the subconscious mind chooses to correlate with the event creates an anchor.

SENSE	POSSIBLE ANCHOR
Sight/Visual	Colors, objects, light, darkness, a person's face, body, body language
Smell/Olfactory	Perfume, food cooking, fresh air, pine trees, exhaust, toxic fumes, incense
Hearing/Auditory	Old song, child's laughter or crying, a person's voice, foghorn, wind chimes
Taste/Gustatory	Mother's cookies, apple pie, roasting turkey, hamburgers, something that made one sick
Feeling/Kinesthetic	Specific place one was touched, hit, or caressed, or a sense of abandonment, betrayal, love

By these examples, if your mind races back to a pleasant childhood memory when you bite into a particular food, it would be stated that you have a positive anchor with that food. If, when you hear a foghorn blowing, it sadly reminds you of your uncle who was lost at sea, you have a negative anchor with that sound. These types of anchors can occur naturally in the course of a person's life.

We can use that same natural ability to our advantage. We can condition positive responses to stimuli. This is done by incorporating anchors into any interaction with another human being—or with a pet, for that matter. Notice the similarity between anchors and Pavlov's conditioning techniques.

Purposeful Anchors

In hypnosis, typical anchors might include touching the client on the hand, forearm, elbow, shoulder, or knee. We can also create visual anchors by suggesting that every time the client sees a color—for instance, red—they will associate that color with a pleasant or empowering sense. These involve environmentally imposed anchors to create a response in the client.

An anchor could be created that involves the client making a certain motion, such as pressing two fingers together, touching a door knob, walking through a doorway, or rubbing their hands together. These are self-generated anchors conjured at will, to enhance self-esteem, confidence, and other desired internal feelings.

A negative anchor may be placed on a person by accident or on purpose. After engaging in an argument with your spouse while they are wearing a red shirt, you may experience an anger response the next time you see them in that shirt, even though the previous argument has long been resolved.

In aversion therapy, an anchor could bind a negative response to the smell of cigarette smoke or the taste of chocolate, in an effort to eliminate undesired habits.

Make It Memorable

The most effective anchors will be those attached to highly emotionally charged experiences. The greater the number of senses involved, the greater the impact of the anchor.

There is a belief that thoughts form clusters of

> **Intensity and multiplicity of sensory experience are vital to creating successful anchors.**

associated material. When we take in an experience, it is filed away in our minds, connected to related stimuli and data. The larger the cluster, the more associated data that is attached, the easier it will be recalled later.

For instance, if, during the course of an uneventful day, you have an unremarkable meal, chances are years later you will have no accessible memory of that experience. On the other hand, when you have an extraordinary meal, with special guests at a unique restaurant to celebrate a special occasion, memories of that meal may be easily recalled at will. This is due to the event having a cluster of stimuli and data connected to it.

Steps to Create an Anchor

By following these steps, you can implant positive, purposeful anchors for your clients.

1. Request the client's permission to touch them on the location of the proposed anchor.

2. Ask the client to recall a highly charged event—one containing the memories that will stimulate the emotions that are desired.

3. During the recall, when the client achieves the greatest connection with the emotions involved, implant the anchor by touching the client in the preordained location, such as on the hand, wrist, arm, or knee.

Sample Script

The following is an example of creating a self-administered anchor when more confidence is desired.

"I wonder if you can recall a time when you felt very confident. A time when you were self-assured and could easily speak with anyone. Recall that event completely, connecting with the sensations in your body and your emotions. Do you recall that event now? Very good. Start at the beginning of the event and move through it, experiencing it fully . . . and tell me when you come to the end of that event. Very good. Start at the beginning of the event once again, and this time amplify the feelings you have of confidence and self-assurance. Connect with those feelings fully in body, mind, and spirit."

As the client achieves this, touch them on the arm, or apply some other anchor that you have agreed upon. Then conclude:

"Anytime in the future when you wish to experience this same feeling of confidence and self-assurance, simply touch your arm here."

Collapsing Anchors

It is possible to bring an element of strength to a client while addressing a negative experience. To do this, first anchor the negative experience in one location. Then, anchor the positive strength in another location. When this has been accomplished, the hypnotherapist can then touch the anchor for the negative experience and immediately touch the anchor for the positive strength, thereby combining these two experiences.

To ensure success, it is wise to anchor the negative event, anchor the positive the event, and then break state. As has been stated before, breaking state is simply a matter of momentarily changing the subject. Test the negative anchor by touching it. Ask the client how they feel when you do this. It is expected that they will answer with words that describe the event, or the emotions involved with that event. If this is not the case, then the anchor must be applied once again, more robustly.

When the testing proves that the anchor is in place, then proceed to test the other anchor for the positive strength. Be certain that the client describes correlating positive feelings when this anchor is touched.

Once both anchors have been tested and proven to be working properly, you may proceed to touch the anchors simultaneously. In this way, the positive strengths have been inserted into the negative event. Upon completion, ask the client how they now feel about that past event. Their response should indicate that they have greater confidence in their ability to handle it.

Notes on Anchoring

A positive anchor provides reinforcement of the client's will and enthusiasm for achieving their goals. It gives them the sense that what they deemed impossible is now achievable. They become assured of their ability to feel and act in this new manner. They give themselves permission to be what they always wanted to be—and are truly capable of being.

> **Anchors are powerful means for instilling in your client, or in yourself, those traits and resources that would be helpful in the course of life's events.**

Installing powerful resources in a client at the beginning of a session will allow them to process painful or frightening memories more successfully. When a client is in the midst of a session and spontaneously encounters something they were not prepared for, it is perfectly acceptable to break from the initial technique and install strengthening anchors before proceeding.

Be conscious of the casual anchors that may be installed by accident. For instance, if you touch a client's elbow when they first arrive in your office, confused or depressed, using the same spot later for a positive anchor will send a conflicting message.

CHAPTER 34

The Empowerment Symbol

The Empowerment Symbol can be exquisitely incorporated into many therapy sessions. When used alone, it is an effective tool for strengthening any desired

> **When the symbol is a small object, such as a stone, many clients seek to obtain one that they can actually hold or carry with them.**

trait. It is also supportive in anchoring desired characteristics in the midst of other therapy techniques. The Empowerment Symbol works elegantly within Outcome therapies, Inner Child work, and any others that benefit from the enhancement of desired traits.

The purpose of the Empowerment Symbol is to take anchoring even further, by asking the subconscious mind to create a metaphor, or symbol, which represents the desired characteristic or feeling.

The idea of the Empowerment Symbol developed when it was naturally produced during a session in my office. The client had conjured a strong positive emotional response that was appropriate to anchor as a gift and future resource. This has since become a useful and versatile contribution to the practice of hypnotherapy.

The Empowerment Symbol delivers an added bonus because it removes the need to touch a client. It may also be more effective for visually oriented clients than the Circle of Excellence, presented in the next chapter, which tends toward kinesthetic access.

Creating the Empowerment Symbol

To produce an Empowerment Symbol, one would simply follow the steps delineated previously for an anchor. Once the desired sensation is thoroughly experienced in the client's body, instead of touching the client, request the Empowerment Symbol.

1. Determine the trait desired by the client.

2. Instruct the client to remember a time when they have experienced this before.

3. Direct them to enhance this feeling using submodalities.

4. Ask the client's subconscious mind to produce a symbol, a metaphor, that represents this feeling.

5. Instruct them to describe the symbol, including its weight, size, texture, and color.

6. Facilitate regression and/or future pacing with the client while they hold the symbol, to discover how possession of the symbol will alter perceptions of various events, past and future.

Sample Script

The following is a method by which the Empowerment Symbol may be elicited. Lead the client through a selected induction, and then continue:

"I invite you to think back over your life, going back to a time when you experienced courage, confidence, and strong self-esteem. Go back to a time when you felt capable of accomplishing your goals. Just nod when you have arrived at that memory. (Client nods.) *Very good. Now, allow yourself to simply move through that experience. Relive those memories, including all the emotions associated with that event. Just give me a nod when you have finished.* (Client nods.) *Very good.*

"Now, go back to the beginning of that event once again. Move through that memory once more, this time stopping at that point in the memory when you are experiencing the greatest sense of that courage, confidence, and self-esteem. When you arrive at that moment, simply nod. (Client nods.)

"Fully experience those sensations of courage, confidence, and self-esteem. Allow them to amplify and fill your body, your mind, your emotions, your energy field, and your very soul. That's right, just feeling those good sensations.

"Now, I would like to ask the subconscious mind to create for you a symbol, a metaphor, that you can imagine holding in your hand, which will represent these good feelings of courage, confidence, and self-esteem. When you see that symbol in your mind's eye, simply nod once again.

(Client nods.) *Describe, please, the symbol that has been presented to you.* (Client describes the symbol.)

"What do you notice about its color? What do you notice about its weight? What is the texture and size of this symbol? What else do you notice about this symbol as you hold it there in your hand? (Pause after each question for your client's response.)

"Now, holding your symbol in your hand, go back in time to a recent event when you really could have used some more courage, confidence, and self-esteem. Do you remember that event? (Client nods.) *Describe what you notice about that event now, moving through it with your Empowerment Symbol.* (Pause for client response.) *In what way does that now seem different from the way you previously remembered that event?*

"Now, please go back to another recent event when you could have used the assistance of the Empowerment Symbol and its associated feelings and sensations. Tell me what you remember about that event. (Pause for client response.) *What do you remember now about that event that seems different from before?*

"Now, carrying that Empowerment Symbol with you, imagine an anticipated event in the future. An event that you are expecting to be difficult. It may involve a situation at work, in your personal life, or any event that could be assisted by having additional courage, confidence, and self-esteem. Can you imagine that situation now? (Client nods.) *Very good. What is the situation that you are anticipating?* (Pause for client response.)

"Allow yourself to move through that anticipated event, now, carrying that Empowerment Symbol with you. Describe what you notice about that event as you move through it now. (Pause for client response.)

"Please go back to the beginning of that event once more. Moving through that anticipated event once again, what do you notice happening this time? (Pause for client response.) *Very good.*

"You know that this Empowerment Symbol is yours. It always has been and always will be. It is yours to use anytime you wish to connect with your own innate sense of courage, confidence, and self-esteem. Use it whenever you want to bolster these good feelings and sensations."

End the session by whatever means are appropriate for that client and that session.

Practice this sequence in your mind until the procedure flows naturally without the use of a script. There will be many opportunities to spontaneously interject the Empowerment Symbol into a session. This will produce a lifelong gift for the client.

CHAPTER 35

The Circle of Excellence

This fascinating therapy technique instills traits of excellence in your client. It allows the client to describe and define their perceptions of excellence and then to "slip into" those very traits. The Circle of Excellence is especially effective for those clients who are more prone to being kinesthetic—those who will benefit from a more sensual experience of the anchor.

Be warned that the Circle of Excellence involves the client standing and walking. Be certain there is an open and clear space in which they may move around.

Sample Script

After achieving hypnosis with your client, use a script similar to the following:

"There is a part of your subconscious mind that knows full well how to remain in this deep state of trance or hypnosis. At the same time, a part of you will find it completely comfortable and very easy to open your eyes. Very good, your eyes are open and yet you remain in this deep trance state. You'll also find it very easy to slowly stand up. That's right. Stand up.

"Watch as I draw an imaginary circle in the center of the room. Observe as I show you this circle now. That's right, the Circle of Excellence is right here in the center of this room. Right in this circle that has been drawn for you, in the center of the room. Imagine, now, that within this Circle of Excellence there is contained every aspect of excellence. Every trait that

you connect with the idea of excellence is contained in this circle. See it now. Feel it. That's right. Very good.

"Now, as I count from three to one, you will step into this Circle of Excellence. Three, two, one. Stepping in. That's right. Very good.

"Notice how you feel there in the Circle of Excellence. Notice your energy. Observe how you stand, walk, move around. Notice your thoughts and emotions.

"Now, as I count from three to one, you will step out of the Circle of Excellence. Three, two, one. Very good. Notice how you feel now.

"Once again, as I count from three to one, you will step into the Circle of Excellence. Three, two, one. That's right. Very good. What do you notice now?"

As the facilitator, observe the changes in the client's posture, countenance, emotions, and movement as they move in and out of the circle.

"Once again, as I count from three to one, you will step out of this Circle of Excellence. Three, two, one. Very good. What do you notice now?

"As I count again from three to one, you will step back into the Circle of Excellence. Three, two, one. That's right, very good. Describe what that experience is for you now.

"You now have the opportunity to bring with you any and all of the traits you are experiencing. Incorporate them into who you are as you step out of the circle. Three, two, one.

"Very good. From this moment on, you will find it easy to maintain this good sensation of excellence. You own it, and you know that it already is an essential part of you. You may now go back to your chair and sit down, while sensing the excellence that you now embody. Very good.

"Once again, I would like you to gently close your eyes. Enjoy this deep sense of relaxation, combined with your experience of excellence. Very good. What do you imagine will be different now that you have regained your sense of excellence?"

Proceed with any further pertinent questions, and then lead the client through future pacing.

The Circle of Excellence is an effective strategy to be used whenever a client needs or desires to incorporate positive strengths within. This technique can also be self-administered.

During one session, a client complained that his shyness and fear of rejection prevented him from approaching women at a singles' dance. He imagined creating his own Circle of Excellence that encompassed the whole ballroom. At the next session, he disclosed that during the next event he danced with several of the women and even made a date for coffee with one of them.

CHAPTER 36

Using a Role Model

The Role Model is an excellent anchoring technique that produces strong results in many circumstances. It can be incorporated into any session when the person is creating behavioral changes, adding special characteristics, traits, and strengths, or trying to model after someone whom they admire. It can be used in private or group sessions.

Weight-loss clients will benefit from this technique when they discover how good they will feel after losing the weight. It also helps them to incorporate the better eating and exercise habits of the future, healthier version of themselves.

It can be a powerful strategy against stage fright. By following the techniques of the Role Model, the client can gain the poise, confidence, and attitudes of their favorite professional.

There are endless beneficial ways to incorporate the Role Model into your practice.

Who Is a Role Model?

This technique can be used in two ways:

- The client can use a future personal model, wherein they have already acquired the success, goals, growth, and learning that they now seek.
- The client can use another person, or a cartoon hero or mythological archetype, for their Role Model, emulating their attitudes, characteristics, or skills.

Role Model Facilitation

In setting up the technique, choose which of the above ways would be the most appropriate for achieving the goal of the therapy session. When using a more perfected version of the client:

1. Ask the client to imagine the future when they have already achieved their goals. They are to imagine that future when they have already gained the desired knowledge and skills or removed the unwanted behaviors.

2. Ask them to look at that future person. Instruct them to notice how they look and move. Ask them to observe their energy and anything else about them.

3. Instruct them to step into that future body on the count of three.

4. Ask them to describe what it is like to be inside that body.

5. Instruct them to step out of that future body and back into their own present body here, at the count of three.

6. Ask them to describe what it is like to be back in their present body.

7. Have them step "in" and "out" several times, each time describing the sensations and perspective they observe. It may also be helpful to have them describe the qualitative differences between the two bodies.

8. When they begin to state that there is little difference, or that they don't want to step back out of that body, the technique can be completed. Alternatively, it can be suggested that they bring desirable traits into their present body.

9. Finish with suggestions that reinforce their ability to remain in this frame of mind, perspective, or sense of being, into the future, as they choose. Remind them that anytime that they feel they have "slipped out" of that desired sense of being, they simply have to remember what it is like, by closing their eyes and once again imagining it.

The same steps will be followed when the client chooses to emulate another person. They will begin by identifying the person or archetype who embodies the traits they desire. If the client is unable to name a role model, they can also create an imaginary person.

Practice Often

Instruct clients on the benefits of spending a few moments every morning upon awakening, and every evening before falling asleep, making sure that they are securely in that new, desired sense of being. They can also monitor that condition throughout the day as needed.

The old adage "fake it 'til you make it" really rings true in this case. When a person practices long enough, the new traits will simply become part of their new persona.

CHAPTER 37

Time Line Therapies

The Time Line is an imaginary visualization of a chronological line, along which are all the perceived events of a life, real or imagined. Many people have developed theories and visualization techniques for moving along the time line. The objective may be future pacing, a modification of Chair Therapy, or simply to facilitate imaginary movement forward and backward along the clients' perceptions of their lives.

The Nature of Memory

Memories of our lives are mostly perceptions of reality, not reality itself. All experiences have been filtered through our "colored glasses," warped by emotions, trauma, inattention, forgetfulness, opinions and influence of other people, as well as many other circumstances.

In hypnotherapy, we are typically attempting to create a new perception for the client that is healthier and happier—one that is more conducive to the positive progress of the client's consciousness and existence. Time Line therapy is one of the tools we can use to achieve this.

When to Use Time Line Therapies

In some cases, Time Line therapy can assist the client in discovering the moment of the onset of a condition, or locating when a "part" first appeared.

Most typically, these techniques are used at the end of a session or as a final session with a client. Apply them after healing has taken place, habits are released or are under control, and objectives have been accomplished.

In this way, traveling along the Time Line allows us to install the present learning and healing into the future and the past.

Monologue or Dialogue

Time Line therapy can be applied as a creative visualization, guiding the client through it without their verbal interaction. Conversely, this tool can involve considerable dialogue, allowing the client to describe what they are experiencing. By including dialogue, various therapies can be applied where needed within the experience. Either way, remember to keep your language nonleading and client centered.

Sample Script

This technique is generally used after other therapies are completed, which have initiated a healing of a disorder, created a preferable behavior, and allowed the client to gain a new sense of themselves. The following script includes one visit to the past and two to the future. Feel free to adjust your own script to provide optimal healing for your client.

"I wonder if you can imagine yourself floating up off of this chair. Floating higher and releasing yourself from time and space. As you lift up out of this chair, you float up through the blue, blue sky, past the white fluffy clouds. You continue floating up through the dark, dark skies and the stars. Floating higher, releasing, until you come out into deep, dark space. So relaxed . . . and feeling so good about yourself.

"As you begin to experience this deep, dark space, this infinite realm, you begin to notice a line, a ribbon, which represents time, and your existence. In one direction that time line moves towards the future, and in the other direction it moves toward the past.

"Some people may experience the line going from left to right or right to left. And others experience it from behind them to in front of them, or vice versa. This particular line can appear in any fashion you so desire.

"This line represents your existence throughout all the moments into the past and all the moments into the future. It represents your existence, your experiences. And, as you begin to move along this line, you begin to notice that there are markers along this line. Each marker represents events, relevant to your experience that you have had in the past or will have in the future. They may be joyous or challenging. They are simply events along the line of your existence.

"Now, turn your attention towards the future. As you begin to move down along that line, you begin to pass those markers. Remaining neutral, simply an observer, you pass the markers. You may be curious as to what those markers represent to you, yet you are confident that there is a part of your subconscious mind that already knows exactly what each represents. Continuing to move along that future time line until that time in the future when you have already accomplished the goals that we have discussed today. As you approach that time in the future, you find a bright and significant marker. One that stands out as unique.

"As you approach that bright spot on your time line, allow yourself to simply float back down to earth. Pass the dark, dark sky and stars, down past the clouds and the blue, blue sky. Gently float down to earth, finding yourself standing right there in that future place. As you look around, you see that part of you that is already in that future. That part of you that has already accomplished these good things. As you look around and as you observe yourself in the future, you begin to notice many things.

"As you observe your future self, notice the way that you move, your posture, and your attitude. As you continue to explore your surroundings, observe the situation in which you find yourself. As you look around, you may discover other things as well. Perhaps there are things that surprise you, situations and events that might delight you. What else do you notice about this experience?

"As you look at that person, who is you in the future, they turn and look at you as well. They begin to tell you about their life. Perhaps you ask them questions. What did they do in order to arrive here in this future? What is it that they remember about their journey that would be important for you to know? If they could share their wisdom with you, what is it that they would tell you?

"Now, saying farewell, knowing that you will soon return here in your physical body, allow yourself to float back up off of the earth. Floating up through the blue, blue sky and clouds; floating up through the dark, dark sky and stars; floating high above the world into the deep cosmos.

"Once again noticing the time line, and all of its fascinating markers, begin to move into the past. Move along that time line, observing the markers with detached curiosity, as you move into the past. Move past today's date. Move on into the past, noticing the markers until you find a marker that once again is more brightly lit. A marker that stands out from the rest.

"As you approach it, allow yourself to drift back down to earth once again. Floating down through the dark, dark sky and stars, down through

the blue, blue sky and clouds. Simply floating down to earth. Finding yourself in an event of the past. Yet, this time you are there with the resources that you have gained from the present and future. As you notice your surroundings, and you see yourself much younger, you observe this event. What do you notice happening as you observe this event this time? What do you observe about your younger self? What information could you share with that younger self? What wisdom will they share with you?

"Allow yourself to float up off the earth, away from that past event. Floating up into the blue, blue sky, past the clouds, through the dark, dark sky and past the stars, all the way back up into the deep space. And once again noticing the time line, allow yourself to move further into the past. Moving back into the past, observing the markers with detached curiosity.

"Continue to move into the past until you notice a particular marker, once again brighter or more distinct. As you approach that marker, allow yourself to simply float back down to earth, floating down past the stars in the dark, dark sky. Float past the clouds in the bright blue sky, and once again land on earth. Looking around, you find that younger version of yourself. As you observe that younger self, what is it you begin to notice about them? What do you notice about this event? What resources and wisdom can you give that younger self? What wisdom can they share with you?

"Now floating back up, up above that event, and away from the earth. Float up through the blue, blue sky and past the clouds; float up past the stars in the dark, dark sky. Floating up into deep space and once again noticing the time line. This time, moving into the future, you fly along the time line. As you move into the future once again, you observe the markers with detached curiosity. Simply observing them. Moving into the future, you discover another more distant time that will be helpful and relevant for you to observe. Once again, simply notice the markers until you find one that is brighter or more distinct. As you approach the marker, allow yourself to simply float back down to earth. Floating downwards, past the stars and the dark, dark sky, past the clouds and the blue, blue sky. Simply floating downwards to earth.

"As you look around you once again, notice yourself in the future. You notice everything about your appearance, your environment, and the events occurring around you. What do you notice? If that "future you" had wisdom to share, what would they tell you? What will it take to get from where you are now, to where you will be, there, in that future? What resources do you have that will be helpful? What resources do they have that could assist you? Now, saying goodbye, assuring them that soon you

will be meeting again, allow yourself to float back up off the earth. Floating up through the blue, blue sky, past the clouds. Float up, past the stars and the dark, dark sky, once again finding the time line.

"Move back along the time line, towards the present moment. Move past the markers, observing them with detached curiosity. When you see the marker that represents this present moment, it will be brighter or in some way distinct. As you approach that marker, allow yourself to float back down past the stars in the dark, dark sky. Float down past the clouds in the blue, blue sky. Float down to earth, floating right down into your body sitting here in the chair, having fully returned to the present moment.

"In a moment, I will be counting from one to five, bringing you back to the present moment. Meanwhile I would like to ask your subconscious mind to continue to reveal to the conscious mind more information, deeper understanding, and knowledge that will be helpful in the strengthening and healing process. And now, coming back to the present moment—one, two, three, coming up, four, aware of this time and space, and five, fully alert and aware—and returned to the present moment."

This technique, which is an example of a specific guided imagery, can be administered to clients or utilized during self-hypnosis, to heal, create change, or discover wondrous possibilities.

> **Create a script of your own to use. It may contain many of the same essentials, yet the visual elements will be unique, perhaps tailored to your individual client.**

PART III

Selected Case Studies

The following case studies demonstrate the use of the techniques presented in this book, combining them and moving smoothly from one to the next. Every client is an individual, with unique qualities, experiences, and issues they wish to work on. No two cases will be alike, and no two cases will follow the same pattern or sequence of techniques.

The names of the clients have been changed, yet the dialogues are close representations of what transpired in the sessions.

> **Learn to tailor your sessions to the needs of the individual.**

CHAPTER 38

Case #1: Jeanette

Presenting Issues: Anger, frustration, blocks, being pulled between two facets of her personality

Strategies: Parts Therapy, Secondary Gains, Regression, Chair Therapy, Object Imagery

Jeanette described herself as being pulled between being a "free spirit," which she liked, and a "church lady," which she felt was a block to her life path.

ML: I would like you to close your eyes, taking a deep breath . . . that's right . . . and just allow your body to relax . . . listening to the music . . . relaxing. And you described to me, just moments ago, that you felt pulled between being a free spirit and being blocked by what you call the "church lady." Is that right?

Client: Yes.

ML: I wonder if you can imagine all of the part of you that you call the free spirit migrating to one of your hands . . . and all of the part of you that you call the church lady moving to the other hand. Allow these two parts of you to separate completely so that they in no way intersect or connect. Completely separated. That's right. Which hand contains the part of you that is a free spirit?

Client: The right.

ML: OK. And the church lady part is on the left, correct?

Client: Yes.

ML: Very good. I would like you to fully move into the right hand, the part that is a free spirit. Allowing it to speak, without any interruption from the left hand, what would it like to say?

Client: It wants to be free, open. It sees a sky full of stars. It is vast, beautiful. There is a peace and security there. Happiness.

ML: And moving to the left side, the one that you call the church lady. Without any interruption from the right side, what would the left side have to say?

Client: It's dark, tightening, angry, pushy, old. It wants to have control. It's a strong force. Solid.

ML: Is there anything else?

Client: No.

ML: Moving back to the right side, what would it like to say?

Client: It wants to let go of the control and soar over the trees. To be in the air. It wants to be young, playful, happy. It is powerful. It is freedom.

ML: Is there anything else?

Client: It also needs security and warmth. To know it's OK to fly. It needs security. It just charges in and does things—no question.

ML: What benefit is there to being on this side?

Client: It has the ability to breathe, see everything, not be scared. To feel powerful and loving.

ML: What is the downside of being on this side?

Client: To be alone. I don't know if anyone else can fly. I need to look. I see people below me, but no one with me. The air feels good.

ML: Anything else?

Client: No.

ML: Moving over to the left side, what is happening there, now?

Client: It's dark, and light. Anger. I'm doing something wrong. I see my grandmother. She's very angry and she doesn't see me. But she is angry. She looks at me and doesn't see who I am. She's yelling. She feels she has done a lot for me and I don't appreciate it. I don't understand because I do appreciate it. She doesn't understand who I am.

ML: What else do you notice about this?

Client: Grandma is sad, lonely. She longs for something. I don't know what. Maybe a better marriage. She wants people to see her for who she is and love her. Her shoulders are slumped and tight, brows furrowed together. She has a lot of wrinkles from being angry all the time. She's shaking. She's angry at me—and at a lot of things. Angry and disappointed. She wants her life to be different. I feel ashamed of something. I always feel ashamed. Sometimes it feels like it's about me and Mom. It's about women. Not men. She doesn't have a voice. Women shouldn't speak up. They should be quiet. They are not worth as much. Not meant for opinions. They're not valuable. Boys are valuable.

ML: How do you feel about that concept now?

Client: I'm sad for her. I wish I could show her women are worth something. That she would think I was worth something. And that she is worth something. I wish she could let go and look at the stars. And be happy with the things that she's done. I wish she wasn't jealous of our relationship with Grandpa.

ML: How can you make her feel better?

Client: I can hug her. I'm afraid she will push me away.

ML: Imagine what it would be like if she does hold you.

Client: We cry. She smiles. I feel better. She apologizes. Tells me I'm pretty. Touches my hair and actually sees me. She knows I'm worth something. I can look at her and know she has beautiful eyes. They're not covered by angry tight eyebrows. She is relaxed and it relaxes me. I'm not scared.

ML: What else do you notice?

Client: I feel empty. I'll fill the space with light. It's beautiful, powerful, and strong. We smile at each other. We're holding each other's arms and there is light between us. It warms us. We're in awe of each other.

ML: What happens next?

Client: We're floating. Not high. Just barely. Like feathers. Light comes over us . . . plumes . . . like a fountain. She smiles. It feels very comforting. We're OK. There are others watching us . . . there . . . they don't know why. I see Grandma and she sees me. Others watch like they're at a movie. Grandma looks younger and tall. I'm still smaller, but it feels right. It's OK.

ML: Tell me now, how is the right hand doing?

Client: It feels bigger. It's throbbing, barely. It's strong. It says, "I told you so!" (She smiles.) It's warm. Now it's arching over . . . and connecting to the left hand.

ML: And what is the left hand doing?

Client: It is getting bigger. Not quite as strong as the right. But it doesn't feel dark or angry. They are going back and forth across this arch, like a rainbow. There is a lot of energy. It looks like a ball. It fits both hands. Energetic, vibrating. The tips of the fingers on the right tingle . . . and the index finger of the left. Everything is quieting. I still feel the hands. There is pressure in the palm of my right hand.

ML: What can you tell me about the sensation in your right hand?

Client: It feels like God.

ML: What else do you know?

Client: It says, "I'm here and will be. My hand is in yours." We're flying. The energy is back with both hands, fingers tingly in both hands.

ML: Have these two hands come to an agreement?

Client: Yes.

ML: What is that agreement?

Client: To work together. Hold light together. Light can go out around; it can project further. The right hand wants to do all the work, though. The left feels weaker.

ML: Is there an important job that you could give to the left hand?

Client: It can keep the right hand from falling, dropping on the floor. It balances it. The right side would shatter if it were dropped. The left gets to touch more of the light. The right keeps it balanced, holds it from below. The left moves around the ball of light. It feels so much of it. The left is excited. It's laughing at the right for only having one job. The right doesn't care. It's not angry. It's just happy. The light can project that way. The left can make shapes, but the right has to hold it from the bottom.

ML: So, tell me again the terms of the agreement.

Client: They function differently in life. The left won't be jealous or angry that the right gets to be so free. The left plays too. They can play together. They are not angry with each other anymore. They are happy with their roles. Not a fake happy, but love and admiration for each other.

ML: I would like these two parts, and your two hands, to come together only so quickly as these parts truly integrate with each other. Coming together in agreement . . . unified, holistically . . . that's right . . . working together . . . feeling so good. Very good. And as these two parts integrate, bring that sense of unity into your body, your mind, your heart, and your very soul. That's right. Feeling so good. . . . So balanced. And how does that feel?

Client: Wonderful! My mind is feeling good. My heart is full.

ML: When you think about the issues that used to make you angry, what do you notice now?

Client: They don't seem so important. I'm not so frustrated.

After further dialogue, the session was brought to closure. Notice that the two sides began to integrate on their own. It is still important to ask the client to verbalize the agreement and to facilitate a formal integration. This reinforces the unification and brings closure to the procedure.

CHAPTER 39

Case #2: Tanya

Presenting Issues: Smoking cessation, self-esteem

Strategies: Hallway Deepening, Parts Therapy, Regression, Inner Child, Role Model, Empowerment Symbol, Future Pacing, Outcome Techniques

In the beginning of our session, the client, Tanya, admitted that smoking was doing nothing for her anymore. She admitted to smoking a pack a day for fifteen years. We covered Secondary Gains during our presession discussion and then proceeded as follows.

ML: I want you to close your eyes and relax as we continue talking. What makes you feel that you are ready to quit smoking now?

Client: Health concerns. My dad died of lung cancer last July.

ML: Have you ever tried to quit before?

Client: Yes, a couple of years ago, but I started up again. Now I have this cough.

ML: What makes this time different?

Client: I want to be more active. I can be if I can breathe better. I want to be here for my great-grandchildren. It stinks and it's expensive. My kids hate it. It's socially unacceptable. I'm tired of the addiction. And the busy-ness in my head. All day I have to think about my next cigarette, go to the bank so I have the money . . . all that.

ML: On a scale of one to ten, ten being the most, how would you rate your motivation to quit this time?

Client: Eight.

ML: What keeps you from being 100 percent motivated?

Client: I'm nervous. When I quit, I think about it all the time. I'm more obsessed than when I am smoking. I'll get uncomfortable and irritable. I'll tell myself it isn't a good time to quit.

ML: Is there ever a good time?

Client: No. There's never a good time to quit.

ML: Tell me about when you started to smoke.

Client: I started in order to annoy the children's father. He was a smoker. I started when we broke up, fifteen years ago. It was stupid, but I did it.

ML: I would like you to imagine a hallway before you. As you begin to move down this hallway, you begin to notice the texture of the floor covering beneath your feet. And the color of the walls. And there are doorways along this hall. Each one leading to the information that will be most pertinent in understanding that first decision to smoke. As I count from three to one, you will find yourself in front of one of those doors. Three, two, one. And what do you notice about this door?

Client: It's wooden, old fashioned, with a brass handle.

ML: As you open the door and step through, what do you begin to notice?

Client: I see myself being very young—about nineteen or twenty years old. I notice how tired she looks, stressed out.

ML: If you could talk with her, what would you tell her?

Client: I would want to tell her to open her eyes. Be aware of what she has. She has two young kids and she loves them. She's in a relationship with an abusive person. She doesn't believe that she could leave or that she could make it on her own. She feels worthless. She seems surprised that I'd say that.

ML: Why is she surprised?

Client: She doesn't think much of herself. She's surprised that I can see her strength and that I care about her.

ML: What else do you want to discuss with her?

Client: She's going to make decisions without regard to how she will feel about them in the future. She can't see that far ahead. When she looks back, she will regret her decisions that she's making now.

ML: What can you teach her or help her with?

Client: It's been hard. She's in survival mode. She thinks day to day, week to week. She doesn't think about the kids and the future. I want to tell her that she has a bright future and that the kids turn out really well.

ML: Why don't you give her a glimpse of your life now, so that she has an idea about that?

Client: She's amazed at the small things—that she owns a car, owns a home, and has a good job with technical skills she has acquired. There is a peacefulness that she treasures daily.

ML: How does viewing your life change anything in her?

Client: She now has hope. She has some vision for that future. She can see herself in that role. She sees that her painful time will end. That she will find peace, love, and satisfaction in life.

ML: Is there anything else to talk to her about?

Client: I want her to know that I do love her.

ML: How will you show her that?

Client: I hug her. I give her some of my power. I let her know that she's strong and powerful.

ML: Can you give her appreciation for all that she has gone through, and the power, strength, and lessons that she has brought to you?

Client: OK. She feels happy. She's astonished. There is a weight lifted. She sees the future and herself in that future. She knows that she can be proud of herself and that it is OK to be that.

ML: Can you give her a metaphorical gift, something that will represent to her the power and wisdom that you are sharing with her today?

Client: Yes, it is a crystal vase of red, fragrant roses. I give it to her.

ML: How does that make her feel?

Client: She's very honored. She feels worthwhile now.

ML: How will what we have done today change her path?

Client: She enjoys and appreciates her children more. She knows how quickly they will grow up. She is now wanting to make some decisions about the party lifestyle—the drinking, smoking, and the occasional drugs. The fast crowd. She is not so willing to do self-destructive things. She cares more about values, family, and the future. She's not as confused about what she wants and what it will take to accomplish that. The glamor of the fast life has worn off for her.

ML: When is the next time that she needs some help from you?

Client: When she is twenty-five years old.

ML: What is going on then?

Client: She's achieved a lot but still needs more self-esteem.

ML: What is going on?

Client: She's in a relationship and not asking for what she wants or needs. She needs to be strong enough to make the decision of asking for changes, or to end it.

ML: What can you do to help her?

Client: I want her to not delude herself. See the signs that are there but she is ignoring. I need to let her know that she's good and she's strong. If she loses the relationship, it could possibly open up better things for her.

ML: Does she accept what you are saying?

Client: She sees that the things I've pointed out are true, but she hadn't brought them to light yet. She is glad to have them confirmed by me. To know that her secret and private thoughts are close to the mark. I tell her to trust her intuition—that it is better than she thinks.

Client: Does she hear you?

ML: She recognizes how many times she intuitively knew but talked herself out of it. I tell her to keep trusting it. The more she does, the stronger it will get for her.

ML: Is there anything else you would like to tell her?

Client: No. She is laughing. She is happy to have things confirmed. To have someone tell her that things are true and right for her.

ML: In what way will this conversation with her change what she does in the future?

Client: I expect that this relationship that she's in will end sooner than it did. She's OK with that. She's not so preoccupied with those issues. She's more involved with nurturing her kids. She's better at taking care of financial issues and making plans.

ML: When is the next time that she could benefit from a conversation with you?

Client: She's thirty-one or thirty-two years old.

ML: What is going on then?

Client: Many things have unraveled in her relationship. She realizes that it's not what she thought. He won't be a father to the kids; he's not committed to her and the family. She's in a stressful job. She works hard and long hours. It's uncomfortable at home. She prefers to work. She is projecting hostility to everyone she loves. She's depressed and gets into a deep hole.

ML: What can you do to help her?

Client: I can understand what she's going through. It's hard to explain to anyone. She doesn't think they understand how bad she feels all the time. I encourage her to seek counseling earlier. She needs it badly. When it is repressed so long, it comes to the surface with all these other issues.

ML: Does she take advantage of your advice?

Client: It helps. She does feel so alone. So isolated. She needs someone there. Someone who cares about her.

ML: Is there anything else you can do for her at this time?

Client: I have an image of me supporting her, carrying her for a while. She needed my help.

ML: And does that help?

Client: Yes. She's able to come through. She gets past the really sad, dark times, back through to the light side. She's all right. All the stronger for what she had to go through.

ML: Can you give her your appreciation for what she went through to get you to where you are today?

Client: I do. I give her appreciation and acknowledgment. And she acknowledges and returns it in kind. That feels very good.

ML: How is she doing now?

Client: She's all right.

ML: When is the next time that she needs some help from you?

Client: I skip in at intervals. Not for anything major or life changing. Small things.

ML: What do you do for her?

Client: I give her words of encouragement—like when she is dealing with teens. I pop in like a good friend once in a while.

ML: How does that work for her?

Client: It helps. It's good to have someone to reflect thoughts off of. She's encouraged that she's doing a good job. There's someone to point out the good things. In the big scheme, some of the bad things were not that major.

ML: How is she feeling now?

Client: Good, comfortable.

ML: Now I would like you to imagine yourself in the near future. A time when you are a nonsmoker, happy, and balanced and you feel good about all that you have achieved. What do you notice about that time in the near future?

Client: She's active, shopping for nice clothes, cute clothes. She takes long walks, bikes, travels to places. She has the energy and stamina to walk, go up stairs.

ML: What else do you notice about her?

Client: She's not feeling tired or out of breath. Her health is good. She looks nice. Her skin is clear.

ML: Do you notice anything else about her?

Client: She's happy, enjoying life. She plays and keeps up with her granddaughter—and maybe other grandchildren. I know that I'll be around a long time.

ML: In what way could that you in the future help the you of today?

Client: She puts out her hand to me and pulls me out of my rut. She says I can do it—I can reach my goals. It's possible. It's doable. I will reach it. It will take time, but it's OK. I'll be healing myself in the process. Healing my body, changing many aspects at the same time. She says to be patient; it will take time.

ML: What strengths and character traits are you learning now that will be added to her?

Client: Admiration and hope. I can see how far I had to go. I see that I was successful. I feel confident now. I know there are many things that I can accomplish when I set my mind to it.

ML: As I count from three to one, I would like you to step into her body, that body in the future. Three, two, one. What do you notice about that?

Client: The sensation of what it is like to be in that body. I can take a deep breath, and not cough. I feel awake, full of energy. I feel it. It's exciting to look forward to.

ML: Is there anything else that you notice about this?

Client: No. Just that seeing and feeling that is very incredible. It motivates me today.

ML: Stepping back into your own body here . . . three, two, one . . . I would like to ask you to separate that part of you that wants to quit smoking from the part that resists that effort. If you were to put each part on either of your hands, which hand would have the part that wants to quit?

Client: The right.

ML: And the left hand has the part that resists that effort?

Client: Yes.

ML: Please allow yourself to go completely into the right hand, the hand that wants to quit smoking. What do you notice about being on that side?

Client: It is warm, tingly, strong, determined. It wants this.

ML: Come out of that side now and move over to the left side. What are its views of this issue?

Client: It's afraid. It will be giving up a habit, its source of comfort. It wonders what it will do without a cigarette. What will replace those moments? It doesn't want to experience bad withdrawals— or the irritability.

ML: What does the right hand have to say about this?

Client: It will take a while. I'll get used to not smoking. I'll take walks, drink ice water, or call someone on the phone. I'll get used to it.

I didn't smoke before and I had things to do. I will do it again.

ML: What does the left hand say about that?

Client: It hates the anxious feeling when it wants a cigarette bad. How will that feel? What if I try, and fail again?

ML: What would be the worst thing if that happened?

Client: I'll be disappointed in myself. I have looked forward to this. I thought about it a lot. But if I fail, I will have to tell others that I wasn't successful.

ML: You have had a child. When they took their first step, and fell, did they fail? Or was falling just a part of the learning process?

Client: A part of the learning process.

ML: Each time they fell, their brains recalculated what went wrong and what they had to do next. Right?

Client: Right.

ML: It was a part of the process. They tried again and again, more steps each time. So each time they fell, it was just a step closer to success, wasn't it?

Client: Yes.

ML: It's the same way with quitting smoking. Chances are someday you will have another cigarette. And that will be OK. Because you will understand why you are having it, and you will know what you need to do to change that in the future. It will be a milestone on your road to health, rather than a failure. What does your left hand have to say about that?

Client: I see that if I have a failure or a setback, it's not all or nothing. It definitely doesn't mean that I can't try again, and be more successful. It may happen. If I do have another cigarette, it's a minor thing, and I can just continue quitting.

ML: How does the left hand feel about that?

Client: It seems quiet.

ML: When the left hand wants that cigarette, what is its goal?

Client: It gives me a pause, a break.

ML: If you could have that break, completely, the way the left hand wants it, then what would you have that is even more important?

Client: A moment of reflection, to think.

ML: If you could have that moment to reflect and think, fully, the way that you want it, then what would you have that is even more important?

Client: I could work out problems.

ML: If you were to work out problems, completely and fully, the way that you want to, then what would you have that is even more important?

Client: I could have quiet meditation.

ML: If you could have quiet meditation, fully and completely, the way that you want it, then what would you have that is even more important?

Client: It would be like coming home to a comfortable, warm place.

ML: If you could come home and be in that comfortable, warm place, fully as you wish it, then what would you have that is even more important?

Client: I'm there, knowing myself well. It's peaceful, connected.

ML: Imagine turning up the intensity on that feeling, just completely immersed in that sensation. I would like to ask your subconscious mind to present to you a symbol that would represent this good feeling of knowing yourself, peacefulness and connectedness. Three, two, one. What symbol do you notice?

Client: It's a lit candle.

ML: If you were to hold that lit candle in your hand, and bring those feelings of connection, peace, and knowing yourself with you into each and every moment, how would that change the way that you experience quiet meditation?

Client: I'd have it on that level all the time. I'd be centered by that in the midst of all the hectic busy-ness. I'd feel it deep at my center.

ML: If you were to carry that candle, and those feelings of connection, peace, and knowing yourself, into each and every moment of the future, how would that change the way that you experience that moment of reflection and thinking?

Client: I'm not sure. You see it is not that important. I would be doing it as I go along more.

ML: If you were to carry that candle, and those feelings of connection, peace, and knowing yourself into each and every moment of the future, how would that change the way that you experience the need to have a cigarette for a pause or a break?

Client: It wouldn't be urgent for me. If I wanted to I could choose to, but it wouldn't be urgent to have the cigarette or the break.

ML: How does the left hand feel now about the prospects of quitting smoking?

Client: It doesn't feel so frightened. It's not afraid of what will happen.

ML: Are there any other concerns that it has?

Client: It worries about key times to smoke. Like after meals and all.

ML: Imagine, now, that you have just completed a meal. See it; feel it. What do you notice about that experience as you observe it now?

Client: I feel satisfied from the meal. I'm comfortable. You see, a lot of times, smoking is a little pause before the next thing I'm going to do. A pause before I get up and do dishes and all that.

ML: So what does the cigarette really represent?

Client: It's a little space between one activity and the next.

ML: What if it was OK to just take a break? If you just declared that you were going to sit and digest, relax a little?

Client: That would be all right. I wouldn't need the cigarette.

ML: What else could you do instead?

Client: I like to read. I could read for a while or watch a show on TV.

ML: Would anyone object to you doing that?

Client: No.

ML: Imagine doing that this evening after dinner. How does that feel to you?

Client: It feels fine. I could look at the paper. I'd put my feet up and relax a couple of minutes.

ML: What does the left hand say about that?

Client: That's possible. I could do that. It's all right to do that.

ML: Would it agree now to let you quit smoking?

Client: It seems to be OK. I don't sense anxiety or fear as much at all. It's not a big deal really.

ML: Are the left and right hands willing to come to an agreement about quitting smoking?

Client: Yes.

ML: Is there any part of you that objects to this agreement?

Client: No, not that I can feel.

ML: I would like you to bring your two hands together now, only so quickly as these two parts of you fully integrate, coming together. That's right. Coming together in unison, moving towards the same goal, towards your health, vitality, and well being. Bringing that integration, now, into your body, your heart, your mind, and your very soul. That's right. And how does that feel now?

Client: I can do this. My body is telling me, "Stop, please stop!"

ML: Do you want to stop the session?

Client: No, I want to stop smoking!

ML: I wonder if you can imagine a future Tanya, the Tanya that is already smoke free. She has successfully given up cigarettes. What do you notice about her as you see her there before you?

Client: She's healthy, strong, physically in good shape.

ML: Do you notice anything else about her?

Client: She's smiling, happy, and confident.

ML: As I count from three to one, I want you to step into her body. Three, two, one. What do you notice about being in her body?

Client: Energy is coursing through me. I can take deep breaths. I'm not coughing. I feel good about myself.

ML: Do you notice anything else?

Client: When I look in the mirror, I'm happy with what I see. My actions, what I do—I'm happy with that.

ML: As I count from three to one, step back out of her and into your own body. Three, two, one . . . stepping out. What do you notice about being back here?

Client: I'm less energetic, more sluggish. I feel weighted down. I have congestion in my chest. My throat is sore.

ML: Stepping back in, three, two, one. What do you notice this time?

Client: I'm so much lighter. I could jump up and go for a quick jog around the park. I could do things in the garden and around the house. I have energy to do them. I feel good.

ML: Stepping back out, three, two, one. What do you notice this time?

Client: I have little aches and pains I didn't have before. And again, my throat is scratchy and sore.

ML: Stepping back into her body, three, two, one. What do you notice this time?

Client: It feels good in this body. It's comfortable, strong. The body is in good shape. It's more flexible. I can stretch. I'm energized.

ML: I wonder if you are curious how you can feel these things while still in this time and space, in this body here. By just using your imagination. As I count from three to one, stepping back out. Three, two, one. What do you notice this time?

Client: I don't think it has changed much. I still feel really energized. The energy is running through my body. I'm relaxed, calm, and confident. It feels good.

ML: And stepping back in . . . three, two, one. How does it feel this time?

Client: I haven't changed much. My throat is not bothering me. I imagine a smaller size of me. That's OK. I'm working on that. I'm OK with who I am until I can get to where I want to be at some point.

ML: And stepping back out, three, two, one. What do you notice this time?

Client: It's the same. I feel very good. There's warmth, tingling. I'm full of energy right now. Excited! I'm looking forward to getting on with life.

ML: Would there be anything else that might prevent you from doing that?

Client: No blocks that I can think of.

ML: In a few moments you will be leaving here and going to your next destination. What do you imagine will happen during the rest of your day?

Client: I'll feel relaxed, calm. I'm just going to have a really good rest of my day. I will see different family members. I look forward to that. I'm jazzed!

ML: Could you spend a moment each day acknowledging your accomplishments? A moment to reflect each day on the good things in your life?

Client: Yes, I can give myself a pat on the back every day. I'll reflect on what I did well each day—another day without smoking. I'll follow my diet plan, exercise. If there are pitfalls I'll recognize that it's nothing and move on.

ML: You said that you were smoking about a pack of cigarettes a day. That is about twenty. Correct?

Client: Yes.

ML: And if you were to smoke each one, not just light it and put it in the ashtray, but really smoke each one, you would have been smoking about two hundred minutes a day, correct?

Client: Yes.

ML: Well, that's about three hours and thirty minutes out of your day, which represents about 15 percent of your day. You spend over twenty hours not smoking! So, we are talking about a very small percentage of your day here.

Client: I never thought about it that way! That is encouraging. It's not as big a thing in my life as I thought it was! This won't be too hard! Thank you.

The session was concluded and the client emerged from hypnosis. Notice the procession from one technique to the next. The client's responses determine the direction and the speed of the session, while the hypnotherapist provides the techniques that will structure the process to achieve the desired goal.

CHAPTER 40

Case #3: Maria

Presenting Issues: Headaches, hypervigilant in sessions

Strategies: Dave Elman Induction, Analytical Imp, Ideomotor and Ideosensory Signals, Reverse Metaphor, Role Model, Secondary Gains, Regression, Inner Child, Personality Part Retrieval, Outcomes

Maria arrived in the office suffering from a headache. She explained that she had suffered from headaches throughout her life. They typically would last about three days. She would experience being sick to her stomach, and nothing her doctors had offered seemed to give much relief. During the pretalk for this session, she also revealed that in her previous session she found herself trying too hard, which prevented the information from flowing as smoothly as it could.

Once again, this session demonstrates a variety of techniques, used in combination, to achieve the desired results.

After facilitating the Dave Elman Induction, the session proceeds with instructions to the Analytical Imp to step aside for the duration of the session.

ML: I understand that there is a subconscious part of your mind that is hypervigilant, which sees its job as one of analysis. I would like to communicate directly with that part of your subconscious mind. In doing so, I would like to ask that part to use Maria's right index finger to indicate a yes response and her left index finger to indicate a no, n-o, response. Moving those fingers, as appropriate, in a fully subconscious manner, with no conscious control of the response. If that is satisfactory, please make your indication to me now.

Client raises right index finger.

ML: Very good. I know that this part of the mind that has been so vigilant and analytical has been very successful in providing safety and survival for Maria. We appreciate all that it has accomplished. It has served a very important role. I am wondering if that part would now like to have an even more important job. Please indicate yes or no.

Client raises right index finger.

ML: Very good. I would like the analytical part to step aside for the duration of this session. To sit up on Maria's left shoulder and observe all that occurs in this session, so that we can confer with it at the end of the session, gaining its insights and observations. Would that be satisfactory? Yes or no?

Client raises right index finger.

ML: Very good. Please move up to the left shoulder now, so that you can quietly observe all that takes place, without interfering in any way, so that you can give us your valuable insights at the end of the session. Just let me know when that has taken place.

Client: OK.

ML: As silly or irrational as it may seem, what does having headaches allow you to do?

Client: They allow me to slow down. They allow me to focus on the headache. And rest.

ML: What does having headaches prevent you from doing?

Client: They prevent me from doing any energetic tasks, or eating well, or enjoying myself. And they keep me from focusing on many other things.

ML: If you were to stop having the headaches, what would that allow you to do?

Client: Everything.

ML: If you were to stop having the headaches, what would that prevent you from doing?

Client: It would prevent me from focusing on the headaches.

ML: I would like to assure that part of your subconscious mind that has created these headaches that we understand that it has been doing this because, in some way, it is trying to communicate a message, and its needs, to the conscious mind. I would like to set up communication with that part of your subconscious mind that has created the headaches, so that we may more fully understand its needs, and thereby find ways of satisfying it without the necessity of the headaches. I would like the subconscious part of the mind that is creating the headaches to produce a signal that will be evident to Maria, or to me, that will indicate a yes, or positive response to a question. Perhaps you will choose to use the fingers of her hands, or perhaps you will choose to intensify or diminish the headache . . . or some other signal you prefer. Please demonstrate the signal for yes, now.

Client: I see a lot of colored lights to the right side of my eyes.

ML: Good. I would like that part of the subconscious mind that is producing the headaches to demonstrate a signal for the no, or negative response.

Client: I see a lot of colored lights to the left side of my eyes.

ML: Once again demonstrate a yes response

Client: I see the colored lights on my right.

ML: And once again, demonstrate the no response.

Client: I see the colored lights on my left.

ML: Very good. I would like to ask that part of the subconscious mind if the headaches are based on a physical cause.

Client: The lights are on the left side. [No.]

ML: Are the headaches based on an emotional cause?

Client: The lights are on the right now. [Yes.]

ML: Are the headaches based on a spiritual cause?

Client: The lights are on the right now. [Yes.]

ML: Are the emotional causes involved with issues of abandonment? [The client had mentioned issues of abandonment and sadness during the pretalk.]

Client: The lights are on the left side. [No.]

ML: Are the emotional causes involved with sadness?

Client: The lights are on the right now. [Yes.]

ML: Are there other emotions involved with the causes of the headaches?

Client: The lights are on the left. [No.]

ML: Do the spiritual causes that you indicate have to do with Maria's sense of God?

Client: The lights are on the right side. [Yes.]

ML: Do the spiritual causes have to do with negative spiritual influences?

Client: The lights are on the left. [No.]

ML: Are there other spiritual causes involved with the headaches?

Client: The lights are on the right. [Yes.]

ML: Is this part of the subconscious mind willing to divulge to the conscious mind what other spiritual causes you are referring to?

Client: The lights are on the right. [Yes.]

ML: As I count from three to one, your conscious mind will under-
        stand the message of the subconscious mind. Three, two, one.
        What is it that you are experiencing?

Client: My eyes feel moister.

ML: What does that indicate to you?

Client: I have a dry-eye syndrome . . . condition.

ML: Is there a connection between the spiritual issues, the headaches,
        and the dry-eye syndrome? Yes or no?

Client: I see the lights on the right side. [Yes.]

ML: I would like the subconscious mind to create for Maria a
        metaphor, a story, that will communicate to us its message con-
        cerning the connection between these issues. We may not know
        where this story begins or ends, or what happens in between, sim-
        ply allowing the story to unfold before us as we move through it.
        As I count from three to one, the subconscious can begin the story.
        Three, two, one. Does your story begin indoors or outdoors?

Client: Outdoors.

ML: Is it day or night?

Client: Day.

ML: What do you begin to notice in your environment?

Client: It's green. There is a tree. It is tall and broad.

ML: What happens next?

Client: I touch the tree. I reach up and touch it.

ML: What else do you notice about that experience?

Client: How immense and large that tree is.

ML: Then what happens?

Client: I start to dance. It feels so free. I am twirling. I am so happy. And now I have tears.

ML: What has created the tears?

Client: Because I don't know if I can be that happy. And now it seems to be getting darker.

ML: What has caused it to get darker?

Client: It's related to my mood. I want to feel happy but don't know how. So, I go to sleep.

ML: Is there anything else that happens in the story?

Client: No.

ML: If the story was a metaphor for experiences in your life here, what would the tree symbolize?

Client: It is life's abundance. When I am happy I can see it.

ML: And then, you reach up to the tree and touch it. What does that indicate?

Client: The feeling of being insignificant is not so strong at that time, when I can touch the tree. I am not afraid to try.

ML: Then you notice that it is immense and large. What does that mean?

Client: Hope. It's comforting, strong, old, and stable.

ML: What would that signify in your life?

Client: There is some dim candle of hope that I find sometimes to keep me going.

ML: Where do you find it?

Client: Deep within myself. When I feel that no one else can give me hope, I can sometimes find it.

ML: And then, you say that you dance. What is that in your life here?

Client: Energy, happiness, freedom.

ML: When do you experience that here? How is it manifested in this life?

Client: When I don't feel bogged down by hard emotions and hard times. When I feel I can grow, and move, and expand.

ML: What allows you to do that?

Client: Confidence, inspiration, time available to do those things. When the needs of others are not overpowering my own needs.

ML: You began to form tears. What were the tears about?

Client: The good feelings feel so short lived. The sadness seems more real. There is always a fear that the happiness will go away, and I won't be able to find it again. The sadness is always there.

ML: What would you be sad about?

Client: I'm sad about not getting outside validation. There is no reassurance, no encouragement for what I do.

ML: You stated that it got darker. What was that?

Client: I curl up and wallow in it.

ML: What do you curl up and wallow in, here in this life?

Client: Overwhelming emotion.

ML: You said that then you went to sleep. What does that mean?

Client: I quit. I turn it off.

ML: What do you turn off?

Client: The overwhelming feelings.

ML: How do you turn them off in this life?

Client: Exhaustion. Worry.

ML: If that metaphor had correlations to your headaches, what would you observe about that?

Client: They are a distraction. They are something else to focus on.

ML: If your headaches were in the metaphor, where would they appear?

Client: After I become sad.

ML: When in the metaphor would they go away?

Client: After I paid enough attention to it.

ML: When would that be?

Client: It would be extra misery between the sadness and the sleep.

ML: If the metaphor had correlations to the dry-eye syndrome, what would they be?

Client: Balance.

ML: What does that mean?

Client: The eyes are dry, or they are flooded with tears. There needs to be something in between.

ML: If you found a place in between, what would that be like?

Client: I could dance.

ML: Can you imagine a future Maria in front of you that has found that balance and is dancing?

Client: Yes.

ML: What do you notice about her?

Client: She is on ice skates. Moving freely, smooth and graceful.

ML: As I count from three to one, imagine stepping out of your body and into hers. Three, two, one . . . stepping in. What do you notice about that?

Client: It's nice to have the speed and skill. I have a slight fear of falling. It's exhilarating.

ML: What do you experience emotionally?

Client: I'm taking in the experience. I'm in the present. Carefree. Like a breeze.

ML: How would she react to taking off the skates and going into everyday activities?

Client: She would be slower. More restricted. There is frustration. She's anxious to get back out there on the skates.

ML: As I count from three to one, step back out into your body here. Three, two, one . . . stepping out. What does it feel like to be back in this body?

Client: Less positive. I wish I could feel anxious for the freedom, rather than lamenting the lack I have here.

ML: What else do you notice about being here?

Client: It's still. There are different fears. Of loneliness, of not being happy, of not being able to feel that free.

ML: Stepping back in, three, two, one. What do you notice this time?

Client: I'm lighter. I don't feel as bogged down. There is better separation between work and fun.

ML: Stepping back out again . . . three, two, one. What do you notice this time?

Client: I'm heavier but more hopeful. I'm getting more energetic.

ML: And stepping back in . . . three, two, one. What do you notice about being in there again?

Client: It reminds me of when I was in my corporate job. There were the restrictions of work, but then I could do whatever I wanted. If I could figure out how to feel like that, then the rest of the time won't be so hard. I would be happy.

ML: And what do you think "happy" feels like?

Client: It is warm. There is less doubt. Less insecurity. Laughing. I would be listened to, appreciated. I would be less self-conscious. Not sad and depressed. I would be living in the moment.

ML: Can you feel all those things now? As you imagine them?

Client: I can when I am in her body.

ML: Could you be her and bring those experiences into your body?

Client: Maybe sometimes.

ML: Bring all those good feelings with you as you step out into your own body . . . three, two, one. What would prevent you from feeling that happiness all the time?

Client: Fears, worries that I know will come around.

ML: What purpose do those fears and worries serve for you?

Client: They keep me from being too vulnerable.

ML: Vulnerable to what?

Client: I have to be prepared for loss.

ML: Can you imagine other ways to be prepared other than having fear and worry?

Client: I don't know how to not worry.

ML: Does that other Maria prepare herself by having fear and worries?

Client: I don't think she worries or has fears.

ML: How does she do that?

Client: She is very centered in herself. She has a good sense of herself. And she is strong.

ML: How would it feel if you were like that?

Client: It feels great.

ML: What would having a good sense of your self and being centered allow you to do?

Client: I would not be blindsided by overwhelming emotions. I would have no worry about other people's wants, their judgments. I would not put myself below other people's needs and try so hard to please everyone else.

ML: Why do you do that?

Client: I have done that ever since I was young. My mother's needs always had to be ahead of mine. Now it is everyone's needs. It's the only way to have peace.

ML: Has putting other people's needs ahead of your own gained you that peace that you desire?

Client: Briefly—in their eyes.

ML: What would having that centeredness and sense of self prevent you from doing?

Client: Nothing.

ML: What does not having that centeredness and sense of self allow you to do?

Client: Nothing constructive.

ML: What does not having that centeredness and sense of self prevent you from doing?

Client: It is crippling when there is not a positive outside influence, whose affections I can earn [said with sarcasm].

ML: With this information, go ahead and step back into that other Maria . . . three, two, one. . . . How does that feel now?

Client: It all seems good.

ML: And stepping out again, three, two, one. What do you notice this time?

Client: I would like to figure out how to feel like that.

ML: Can you remember a time when you did have positive self-centeredness? Did you have that as an infant?

Client: I don't ever remember it. It was always being squashed by my mother.

ML: If it was being squashed by your mother, you must have had it. Right? Go back to a time when you were struggling to hang on to it, even though your mother was attempting to squash it. How old were you?

Client: I must have been around five years old.

ML: Allow yourself to go back there . . . getting smaller, younger . . . going back to five years old. What do you notice about that experience?

Client: I was sad and fearful. I kept trying ways to combat it. But everything I tried got beaten down.

ML: If you tried that hard, it must have been something that you really valued. True?

Client: Yes.

ML: As hard as you wanted to hold on to it, as much as you valued it, little by little it began to slip away from you. Perhaps you dropped it; perhaps you hid it carefully. Maybe it just was left somewhere. As you imagine that experience now, if you could imagine that part of you as though it had a shape and a color, as though it were an object of some sort that you lost, what would be its shape and color?

Client: It's like a glowing ball.

ML: Go ahead and search for it. It may have been left on a shelf, on the floor, in the yard, somewhere in your childhood environment. Wherever it was left, locate it now. What do you notice?

Client: It must be a little candle that I can only see sometimes. It hides in the dark. I don't know where to find it. Once in a while, it appears for a little bit.

ML: When it appears, is it in your energy field, or in your childhood environment?

Client: It is in me.

ML: I would like to ask your subconscious mind that has been keeping this energy safely hidden to reveal it to you now. What do you notice?

Client: It is much brighter than the glimpse I usually get.

ML: Does it feel that it is OK to come out of hiding?

Client: Yes.

ML: What would happen if it did?

Client: I would figure out what I want. I could let go of the feelings of things that are inflicted by others. I could feel free and happy.

ML: Is there any part of you that would have objections to this happening?

Client: The part that is a mother, with all the "shoulds" of motherhood.

ML: Can you imagine that what you do for your children could be an act of selfishness? Taking care of them could be a means of making you happy.

Client: It's confusing. I feel I have been doing those things all along, but my feelings were not in line. There has been an urge, a push, to do the things that I have done, but I didn't know where that was coming from. I felt that I needed to do those things or be miserable. I haven't learned to be in it, fully appreciating the changes I've made.

ML: Why don't you take a moment to give yourself that appreciation, now? To really appreciate all that you have been through and all the growth that you have achieved so far?

Client: (Pausing.) That feels good.

ML: Do we need to anchor that candle, that energy of the sense of self and centeredness? Or is it going to be OK the way that it is?

Client: I want to keep it out. It is going to be OK where it is.

ML: I would like to go back to that part that has been producing the headaches. Communicating with that part now, have we addressed the spiritual causes that you indicated in the beginning of the session? Yes or no.

Client: The lights are on the right. [Yes.]

ML: Would you be willing to remove the headaches as long as Maria remains centered and retains her sense of self?

Client: The lights are on the right. [Yes.]

ML: Is there anything else that she will have to do to avoid the headaches?

Client: The lights are on the left. [No.]

ML: Will you be willing to remove the headache now?

Client: The lights are on the right. [Yes.]

ML: Thank you. Go ahead and release the headache now. Relaxing. Now, I would like to ask the analytical part that has been observing this session to come back off Maria's shoulder and reintegrate. All the parts now integrating and uniting as one . . . very good. I would like to ask the analytical part what observations it has had regarding the session.

Client: There's hope.

ML: Would you prefer to remain in your normal body or would you like to stay in that other Maria?

Client: I prefer the new Maria.

ML: Make sure that you are sensing yourself in her body now . . . three, two, one. How does that feel?

Client: Fine. Much better.

We closed the session at this point with a typical emergence technique. Maria disclosed that her headache had significantly reduced in strength. There was just an echo of the original sensation. She was feeling very enthusiastic about the possibilities opening up on her path.

Notice the structure of the yes/no questions. Even when there is a yes response, it is important to continue giving other choices, as there may be more than one causation or answer. Also, observe how the various techniques lead the session down several tangential paths. By the end, closure had to be achieved in each of them. This makes a strong case for the necessity of organized and detailed note taking.

CHAPTER 41

Case #4: Jolene

Presenting Issues: Ulcerative colitis, diarrhea, blocked emotions, lacking personal boundaries

Strategies: Object Imagery, Secondary Gains

Jolene explained that her doctor had diagnosed her with ulcerative colitis. She had been suffering with it for several years and it had flared up once again. Her symptoms included diarrhea and mucous-laden bowels.

After turning on some gentle music, I asked my client to sit back, relax, and take a deep breath.

ML: And as you begin to look inwards, become fully aware of the sensations that you are experiencing in your abdomen. As you continue to observe this area, what do you begin to notice?

Client: It is red, raw. It rejects anything that is going through it. It is sore. It doesn't want anything to touch it.

ML: If those feelings you are describing had a shape and a color, what would you notice about that?

Client: It would be a rock. Like a pebble washed up on the shore. It is smooth around the edges, yet hard and solid. Not giving.

ML: If you could telepathically communicate with this rock, what would it tell you that it is doing there?

Client: It makes me listen. It teaches me.

ML: What is it trying to teach you?

Client: That I can't go through life with blinders. I have to take notice. I can't ignore anything and everything. I can't let things pass through my life without their effects on me. I learned that trait from my father. That if I don't acknowledge it, there is no problem. It's telling me I can't dismiss everything.

ML: Is there anything else?

Client: It doesn't mean that you have to let things get the best of you, but you have to sit up and take notice. It's OK to be more emotional. I have to do more than go through the emotions. I have to feel what I say and do.

ML: What else do you know about that?

Client: I'm the reactionary. If my siblings acted up, I'd be good. If my husband flies off the handle, I become the calm one. Plus, we are not involved in affection. It's a family trait.

ML: What does having that rock there allow you to do?

Client: It is similar to when I gained weight in my teens. I was painfully shy as a child. I was not popular with the boys because of the weight. The colitis is similar. The rock insulates me from the world. I can't be far from the bathroom, and sex is not available. It shelters me from the world and from my husband.

ML: What does having that rock in there prevent you from doing?

Client: It prevents me from opening to my emotions like I should. It is hard for me to even say I love my husband. I haven't had a lot of experience with people who are open with their emotions. It is scary to imagine it.

ML: So now when you look at that area of your abdomen, what do you notice?

Client: The rock goes to my heart and hardens it. And it goes to the digestive system and hardens that. It's the only way to prevent injury—to harden. Then the heart doesn't function well, and then the digestion acts up.

ML: What would you like to do about this?

Client: I need to let go of it so that the body and emotions can heal. If I don't, everything will get harder and harder. It will create more problems.

ML: What can you do to accomplish this?

Client: It turns viscous. It is like a liquid; it begins to flow. It becomes vibrant. The hardness is gone. Underneath is healthy tissue. It feels like it can breathe. It hasn't felt like that for a long time.

ML: How do you feel?

Client: There is relief. It has worked its way out.

This short segment does not indicate a full healing of the symptoms. However, underlying causes were revealed and certain shifts were allowed to take place. Many auxiliary issues were uncovered that will also require attention in future sessions.

CHAPTER 42

Case #5: Joseph

Presenting Issues: Exposure to toxic mold and fungi, forgiveness, shame

Strategies: Chair Therapy, Parts Therapy, Outcomes, Future Pacing, Empowerment Symbol

There had been numerous sessions with this client over a couple of months concerning health issues pursuant to his being exposed to toxic mold and fungus spores. Many positive changes had occurred and the client revealed his need for self-forgiveness around this issue.

Client: It's time for me to forgive the parties involved and myself. I also need to get to a place where I can see the brighter side.

ML: What will it take to forgive the other people involved?

Client: I'm getting closer. I still have the need to be vigilant. I need to be clear before I forgive. It's the recognition of what still needs to be done. I can't forgive in the absence of that.

ML: What would it take to forgive yourself in this matter?

Client: In regard to myself, I'm closer to forgiving.

ML: Would you like to achieve that forgiveness now?

Client: I think I am ready.

ML: Close your eyes, breathe, and visualize an image of yourself, there in front of you. As you imagine yourself there now, what is it that you notice about "that you"?

Client: He is stronger, clearer. He's more self-assured. He has been humbled in a different way. He did the best he could.

ML: Given the information and ability that he had then, could he have done anything different or better?

Client: No, there was nothing else he could have done. It was like he was trying to find his way out of a maze. Or trying to get out of a cave with a failing flashlight, candles, and some wet matches.

ML: What do you need to forgive him for?

Client: He needs forgiveness for not seeing it earlier. For not listening.

ML: What clues would he have had that would have told him to pay attention? What was it he missed?

Client: If he could have known when that catastrophic water damage occurred.

ML: At that time, what clue would he have had that would alert him to the danger?

Client: He should have known about the danger of mold forming. He just couldn't imagine how dangerous it was.

ML: If he couldn't imagine that, why is he being held accountable?

Client: He expected the workers to be more competent. I need to forgive him for his assumption of their quality of work. And for the negligence of the owners. He should have looked more closely at the fine print on the contract. He just couldn't imagine that it would turn out to be important. He didn't realize how they [owners] would hide behind things. He didn't know who to turn to. He certainly has learned important lessons.

ML: Would it be possible for you to give him your appreciation for all that he has gone through? Can you appreciate him for the lessons that he had to go through in order for you to gain the wisdom that you have now?

Client: (Pausing.) OK, I gave him my appreciation. He feels better. Relieved. He feels like a veteran. He's war weary. He suffered so much damage.

ML: Are you able to forgive him now?

Client: For some reason, I am still resisting it. I feel like I am receding, angry and judging.

ML: Would you say that it is true that there is a part of you that wants to forgive yourself, and another part that is resisting that proposal?

Client: Most definitely.

ML: If you were to separate those two parts, so that the part that wants to forgive yourself is resting on one of your hands and the part that resists that effort is on the other hand, which hand has the part that wants to forgive?

Client: The left.

ML: And the right has the part that is resisting?

Client: Yes.

ML: When these two parts are completely separated, and in no way touching or intersecting, please allow yourself to go into the part that wants to forgive. If it were given the opportunity to speak out, without any interruption from the other side, what would it have to say?

Client: It would feel better. It is the right thing to do. I could heal and have closure. It would be streamlined, less of a drag. Not be stuck. It would be right.

ML: Coming out of the left hand, and all the way over to the right hand, if it were to speak, without interruption from the other side, what would it have to say?

Client: He doesn't deserve it. I need to punish him and keep him in his place.

ML: Coming back over to the left side, how would it respond to what it just heard?

Client: I understand. But you don't need to be there. It is the shame that you carry from your father, and his father, and his father. The shame is theirs, and you need to turn it back to them. It doesn't help you.

ML: Returning to the right side, how would it respond to what it just heard?

Client: How will I know where I am if I'm not kept in my place? That shame has fueled me. It has kept me going.

ML: By maintaining this sense of shame, what is it that you want for Joseph? What is the goal of that shame?

Client: It's an anchor. It maintains a connection with my father.

ML: If you were to achieve that anchor fully, exactly the way that you want it, then what would you have that is even more important?

Client: I would have acceptance.

ML: If you were to have acceptance, fully, exactly the way that you imagine it now, then what would you have that is even more important?

Client: Peace. But a terrible peace—like inertia. It would be like a bug stuck on a pin.

ML: If you were to achieve that type of peace, exactly the way that you imagine it now, then what would you have that is even more important?

Client: If I achieved it in the essence of its highest nature, it feels like being crushed.

ML: I would like to ask the right hand if that is its goal. Is that what you want?

Client: The right no longer seeks that. He knows now that he has to change, to shift, and to let go. He feels a sense of responsibility. He feels that the pangs of guilt and anxiety can be motivational and serve as important feedback. But he realizes that he must not get overwhelmed with toxic shame. It was a message from my father— the shaming around who I was and am. It's not fair. It's not right.

ML: What does the left hand have to say now?

Client: There is a much better way. I see it, and you [right hand] must come with me. It will get better.

ML: What does the right hand have to say now?

Client: Reluctantly, I'll follow you. I'll follow, but I'm scared.

ML: What is the right hand scared of?

Client: It's scared of punishment and retribution; afraid of those who would shame him. I realize it is not realistic. I need to shut that door.

ML: Can you do that now?

Client: Yes, I just did.

ML: How does that feel?

Client: It's better. There is a boundary, a limit.

ML: How does the right hand feel now?

Client: Lighter. Much better. It's encouraged, but it needs help.

ML: What does the left hand say about that?

Client: I'll help. Follow me.

ML: Are these two parts willing to work together now?

Client: Yes, they are ready.

ML: Is there any other part that would object to this agreement to work together for these goals?

Client: There's no resistance.

ML: Allow these two hands to come together only so quickly as these two parts combine their energies and integrate. Integrating fully, becoming one, whole. When these two energies have completely merged, allow that energy to come into your body, your heart, your mind, and your very soul. That's right . . . very good. How does that feel?

Client: Great.

ML: I want you to picture Joseph in front of you again. As you look at him now, what is it that you notice?

Client: He is much more calm. He has clarity and peace. There is an understanding now. Less turmoil and conflict.

ML: Would you be able to forgive that man now?

Client: Yes, I forgive him.

ML: Go ahead and tell him you forgive him, silently, to yourself. Just tell me when you are finished.

Client: OK.

ML: I would like you to imagine yourself three months from now. Just go out into the future about three months and observe what is happening then. What is it that you notice?

Client: There is less undermining of myself. I am not so self-deprecating. I'm freed up to focus on where I need to go and the changes that need to be made. I take better care of myself. I pace myself and am more patient. I am enjoying the process. It's good. It is a different part of the adventure. It's exciting. I'm motivated to resolve this issue. I'm a live wire!

So why not anchor that exuberant feeling? I used the Empowerment Symbol to reinforce this feeling. The chapter on the Empowerment Symbol provides further information on this technique. After that, the session was brought to closure. Once the client achieved self-forgiveness, subsequent sessions afforded the opportunity to address forgiveness for others.

CHAPTER 43

Case #6: Lucille

Presenting Issue: Weight loss

Strategies: Secondary Gains, Parts Therapy, Outcomes, Empowerment Symbol, Future Pacing

A client came into the office as part of a weight-loss program designed by the Washington Athletic Club, an exclusive social and athletic organization in Seattle. I provide the hypnosis aspect of their multifaceted Why Weight? Program. She disclosed that she had successfully quit smoking after two sessions with a hypnotherapist, so she was a willing subject, filled with positive anticipation of the outcome of our session.

I will transcribe the beginning of the session to show how other therapy techniques easily lead into the use of outcome therapies.

The session began with Secondary Gains.

ML: What does having this extra weight allow you to do?

Client: Nothing.

ML: What does having this extra weight prevent you from doing?

Client: It makes it harder to exercise. It is bad for my back. I cannot wear the nice clothes in my closet. It affects my cholesterol, my health, and my perception of myself.

ML: What would losing this weight allow you to do?

Client: It would give me more energy, I would enjoy exercising more, and I could stop my cholesterol medication. When I look in the mirror, I would see a person I recognize. I would be healthier.

ML: What would losing this weight prevent you from doing?

Client: I can't think of anything.

ML: Would you say that it is true that there is a part of you that wants to lose this weight and another part of you that resists that effort?

Client: Yes, that is true.

ML: I would like you to separate these two parts of you completely, so that each part is resting on either of your hands. As you do so, which hand has the part that wants to lose the weight?

Client: The right hand.

ML: And the left hand contains the part that resists that, correct?

Client: Yes.

ML: Allow yourself to go into the right hand, the hand that has the part that wants to lose weight. When you have done so completely, allow the right hand to express itself concerning this matter fully and completely, without any interference from the other part. What would it say?

Client: This is something you can do. You have control. You can change. Think how much better you would feel and look.

ML: Now allow yourself to go into the left hand, the hand that has been resisting this effort to lose weight. Without any interference from the right hand, what would this hand have to say about this issue?

Client: But you love to cook; you love to eat; it gives you pleasure. You associate food with friends and good times. Don't deny yourself that. Remember how good it makes you feel. The food brings you comfort.

ML: Moving back to the right hand, what would it say in response to what it just heard?

Client: I just listed the pain that the weight causes me. How can the eating bring comfort?

ML: And what would the left hand say in response to that?

Client: You have such pleasant memories with friends revolving around meals you've shared. You won't be able to cook anymore or share those experiences with your friends.

ML: What would the right hand say about that?

Client: You can still do it. You just have to eat less. You can have everything you want. You can cook; you can go out. Just don't eat everything.

ML: What does the left hand have to say now?

Client: It's stumped.

ML: What does the right hand have to say?

Client: You can do this. You're good at accomplishing your goals.

ML: And what is the left hand saying now?

Client: I'm still going to try to get you.

ML: I would like to ask the left side what its goal is in resisting the weight loss.

Client: It's just this one time so it won't matter. Everyone else is eating dessert.

ML: If you could describe your goal in one or two words, what would you say your goal is in resisting the weight loss?

Client: Acceptance.

ML: If you could achieve acceptance, fully, exactly the way you want it, then what would you want that is even more important?

Client: Power.

ML: If you could achieve power, fully, exactly the way you want it, then what would you have that is even more important?

Client: I would be a partner with the right side.

ML: If you could be a partner with the right side, fully, exactly the way you want it, then what would you have that is even more important?

Client: Peace of mind.

ML: If you could achieve peace of mind, fully, exactly the way you want it, then what would you have that is even more important?

Client: Self-love.

ML: If you could achieve self-love, fully, exactly the way you want it, then what would you have that is even more important?

Client: Happiness.

ML: If you could achieve happiness, fully, exactly the way you wanted it, then what would you have that is even more important?

Client: That's it. That would be the ultimate.

ML: Very good. As you experience that happiness, exactly the way that you imagine it now, I wonder if you can amplify the feeling. Simply turn up the volume. Intensify that wonderful feeling of happiness as you imagine it now. Feel it in your entire body. Feel it in your emotions, your thoughts, and throughout your entire being. As you fully experience this sensation of happiness, I would like to ask your subconscious mind to present to you a symbol that would represent this good feeling of happiness. Perhaps it is a symbol that you could hold in your hand. And as your subconscious mind produces that symbol for you, what is it that you notice?

Client: It's a sun.

ML: You may realize now that you have always had this happiness within you. It has always been a part of your existence, a part of who you are. Now as you experience this happiness, and hold that sun in your hand, you can know that you will have access to this feeling any time you wish. And now, if you were to carry that sun and this sense of happiness with you each and every moment into the future, how would that change your experience of self-love?

Client: I would feel better about myself.

ML: If you were to carry that sun and this sense of happiness with you each and every moment into the future, how would those change your experience of peace of mind?

Client: I wouldn't have to think about this all the time. I could focus my attention on other things.

ML: If you were to carry that sun and the sense of happiness with you each and every moment into the future, how would that change your experience of being partners with the right hand?

Client: I would be able to find new pleasures.

ML: If you were to carry that sun and this sense of happiness with you each and every moment into the future, how would those change your experience of power?

Client: I would already feel like I was in control.

ML: If you were to carry that sun and this sense of happiness with you each and every moment into the future, how would those change your experience of acceptance?

Client: I would have more confidence.

ML: If you were to carry that sun and the sense of happiness with you each and every moment into the future, how would those change your experience of being able to eat dessert like everyone else?

Client: I could just say no. I would be happy with one bite, and leave things on my plate.

ML: And how would that make you feel?

Client: That would be so good. I would feel really good.

ML: What does your left hand have to say now about this issue?

Client: It is emptier. It has less power. It is shrinking.

ML: And what does your right hand have to say now about this issue?

Client: It is stronger. It feels more confident and powerful.

ML: What does your left hand have to say now?

Client: It's smaller.

ML: Is there anything else that it needs in order to agree with the right side?

Client: It needs to experience enjoyment.

ML: In seeking this type of enjoyment, what is its goal?

Client: It wants me to feel good and be happy.

ML: Happy about what?

Client: It wants me to be happy about myself.

ML: Does this part feel that it has been successful in making you happy about yourself through the methods it has used so far?

Client: No, it understands that I have not been happy about myself.

ML: Would it be willing to make a change if a new behavior could achieve the goal it wants for you?

Client: Yes, it would.

ML: What is it that the left hand wants?

Client: It wants me to have good health and energy. It wants me to express myself creatively—through writing, art, music, and learning a language.

ML: If you were to agree to begin to express yourself creatively, how would it feel?

Client: We could do that. It would be satisfied.

ML: And how would the right hand feel about this?

Client: It would love to try these things.

ML: How will the left hand help to initiate these activities?

Client: She already knows how to. She just needs to do it. She needs to make the phone calls.

ML: Have the right and left hands come to an agreement concerning this issue?

Client: Yes.

ML: How would that agreement be stated?

Client: We agreed to look for other ways to be creative—other ways to be social and enjoy friendships. We will move the food issue into the background. We won't focus on it anymore. It will be a smaller part of all our activities.

ML: Allow these two hands to come together only so quickly as these two parts integrate, coming together as one, their energies mingling and combining. Integrating these two parts, fully and completely, allowing them to work together in unison and harmony. And when they have completely integrated, allow that integration to come into your body, your heart, your mind, and your very soul. How does that feel now?

Client: I feel very content. It's wonderful.

ML: Now that these two parts have fully integrated, what do you imagine will be your first steps in initiating this new game plan?

Client: First of all, I will eat smaller portions.

ML: And what else will you do to support your new decision?

Client: I will look for opportunities in socializing that do not involve food, such as hikes, visits to the museum, concerts, classes, and long walks with friends.

ML: Imagine the next time you go out for a meal with your friends. What is it that you notice about that event?

Client: I will focus on the people and the conversation. The food will fade into the background. It feels really right like this. My friends will be the focus. It is more pleasurable. Everything feels good about that evening. I enjoy my friends and am pleased with the focus, which is on the conversation, not the food.

We brought the session to a close with supportive suggestions and an emergence from hypnosis. Notice the client's explicit use of submodalities in describing her internal experiences: smaller, empty, shrinking, fade, stronger, and so forth. This provides the natural opportunity to integrate them into the session.

CHAPTER 44

Case #7: John

Presenting Issues: Self-esteem, confidence

Strategies: Role Model, Chair Therapy, Reframing

John was preparing for an important sales meeting in Saudi Arabia. His confidence had been shaken by recent setbacks. We decided to rehearse for this meeting with hypnosis strategies.

ML: As you close your eyes, breathe, and begin to relax, imagine going into that meeting. You have arrived there in Saudi Arabia, and the meeting is about to begin. What do you notice about that?

Client: There is a lot of excitement in everybody. And a lot of energy.

ML: Whom do you see there?

Client: I see the powerful John. He wanted to make sure he was there, dealing with successful people. The kind I haven't been around before.

ML: What else do you notice?

Client: I am able to grab and challenge them. I earn their respect quickly. That's important.

ML: What do you notice about the interaction?

Client: It feels great! I'm counting on the interaction.

ML: Do you have any concerns about customs or differences between you?

Client: The concerns aren't there regarding roles, dress, or skin differences. I just don't sense that.

ML: What else do you notice?

Client: It's fun! There is enjoyment and laughter.

ML: Move ahead to the end of the meeting. What are you noticing about that?

Client: I feel great affection and appreciation. It has been a meaningful facilitation. There are wonderful feelings. I achieved my goals. There are smiles and laughter.

ML: Is there anything that you would like to change or improve?

Client: There is nothing to change. Get me there! I want the plane to leave today!

ML: Focus, now, on the primary Saudi delegate. In a moment, I am going to ask you to step into his body—your legs in his legs, your arms in his arms, and looking out through his eyes. Now, as I count from three to one, allow yourself to just move right into his body. Three, two, one. What do you notice about being in his body?

Client: He's wondering about me. He feels powerful. He is used to giving orders that are followed. There is a swagger to him.

ML: How does it feel to be in his clothing?

Client: It feels different. They are fine robes, white.

ML: How is he feeling about this encounter with a group of Westerners?

Client: He has his reservations. He feels pushed into this meeting. He's required to do it by his company, his superiors. He had to clear his slate for several days. He feels he doesn't need this meeting. He does OK without it.

ML: How does he feel about the Westerners' behaviors and mannerisms?

Client: He finds humor in them. They are different from his customs.

ML: What are his perceptions of the meeting?

Client: He now sees the value in it. He starts to become engaged. It is not so bad; there is something positive to this. He can't just sit through it. He has to interact.

ML: What else is he thinking?

Client: He is wondering, "Who is this guy? Why listen to him?" My bio will grab him. He will be impressed with all my experience. Then there is the interaction.

ML: When the meeting ends, what is he thinking?

Client: He feels a sense of accomplishment. He knows he got something out of it. He enjoyed the experience. He was impressed by the experience and the interjections.

ML: All right. I would like you to step out of him now. Three, two, one. How are you feeling?

Client: Great! Let's get started! [He rubs his hands together and smiles.]

ML: I wonder if you can imagine that successful John, standing right there in front of you. As you do that, what is it that you notice about him?

Client: He stands upright, he's taller, has high energy. He's almost glowing. He wants to get started.

ML: As I count from three to one, I want you to step into him. Three, two, one. Stepping into that future, successful John. How does that feel?

Client: Oh boy! I'm tingling! There is a knowing—that this will happen. I can do anything.

ML: Now, as I count from three to one, I want you to step out of him and back into your body here. Three, two, one.

Client: It's difficult to get out. In this body, I'm not tingling. But I still feel great.

ML: Going back into that successful John . . . three, two, one. What do you notice this time?

Client: It makes me smile. The tingling has come back. There is such confidence. This is me and it's something I can do.

ML: Coming back out of that body . . . three, two, one.

Client: I'm not coming out. This feels too good.

ML: Is there anything that could get you out?

Client: No. There is no situation and no person that could make me leave here. I like this feeling. They are waiting to hear me speak.

ML: Staying in this body, this perspective, and these feelings, how do you imagine that it will change what you do today?

Client: I had some nuisance work to do today. Now it doesn't feel like such a hassle. I have to go home and lay out my clothes for the trip, and do all those things to get ready. Just odds and ends.

ML: What if you were to view the jobs to be a part of the magic that sets the tone for the entire trip? What if everything you did in preparation was a part of the end result?

Client: That makes me smile—and the tingle is intensifying. If I think about everything I do as magic for what is to follow, there is a lot of energy! That feels great. I'm feeling really centered. I'm a ball of energy!

The session was concluded with anchoring that "ball of energy" and emergence from hypnosis. Notice how the client moved from the mindset of self-doubt to one of full confidence and enthusiasm. All of these perceptions are available to every human being. It is a matter of choice.

CHAPTER 45

Case #8: Roberta

Presenting Issues: Self-esteem, confidence, independence

Strategies: Reverse Metaphor, Object Imagery, Parts Therapy, Empowerment Symbol, Submodalities, Regression, Inner Child, Personality Part Retrieval, Outcomes

Here is an example of how a Reverse Metaphor leads to several other therapy techniques in order to arrive at a resolution for the client. It is sometimes difficult to decipher where the lines exist between metaphor and possible memories of this, or an alternative, life. Just allowing it to flow as the client experiences it heals best. After all, its relevance and meaning is specific to the client.

After the induction and the Hallway Deepening technique with instructions for the subconscious mind to create a metaphor that will help us to understand its message to the client, we proceed:

ML: Describe the door where you are standing.

Client: It is a plain wooden door. It's ordinary, and it's at the end of the hallway.

ML: As you open the door and step through, where does your story begin?

Client: Outdoors. It is desertlike, sandy. It is somewhere I have been before in a session. It seems to be in the Southwest—even Mexico. There is a Southwestern influence on the house construction and the furnishings. It's in the past, but not far.

ML: What else do you notice about this scene?

Client: There are not too many people. I go into the house. It's quiet. There is a woman sitting in an easy chair. She looks like my mother did in her forties or fifties. She is the mistress of the house. She is rooted to her chair. She has a drink and a cigarette.

ML: What else do you notice about her?

Client: She appears to be in a cocoon, dwelling in the past and how unjust her life has been. She is oblivious to everyone, although I'm there and so are a few others. She will talk with us, though she is egocentric. This is the daily routine. Most of the day is spent with her "holding court." She gives orders to the servants, is constantly bemoaning her rough life. Few people can do things right. She is not able or willing to do things for herself. She doesn't want to change it either. Everyone is around her, yet they keep their distance. She is powerful—the boss.

ML: Is there anything else that you notice?

Client: She can be nice, but when she drinks, she becomes negative. I'm her daughter, though I don't live there. I'm on my own. I don't do much of the caretaking.

ML: What else do you notice about this story?

Client: The years pass. The mother is older, and decrepit. I realize that I can't depend on her for anything. I need to become self-sufficient. I want my independence, yet I want her mothering. There is no choice. She loves me though she has no time for me. I feel sorry for her, and for myself. I have forgiven her for the way that she is.

ML: As the time continues to pass, what else do you realize?

Client: I see the determination. It is almost as though she doesn't exist. I was in my midforties when she died. Yet, I lost her long before that. [Client shows slight abreaction.]

ML: What are the emotions that you are experiencing?

Client: Sadness. A defeated feeling. It doesn't matter what I do or say. She won't snap out of the situation. Defeat.

ML: If that sadness and defeat were located somewhere on your body, where would it be?

Client: In the pit of my stomach.

ML: If that sadness and defeat had a shape and a color, what would it look like?

Client: A large ball, the size of a baseball. It would be gray, dead. It could be blocking movement.

ML: If you could separate that part of you that has created this feeling, this ball, this blockage, from the part of you that wants it to be clear, with freedom of movement there . . . if you could separate those two parts of you, so that each part rests completely on one of your hands, which hand would have the ball?

Client: Right.

ML: And the left hand would have the part of you that wants it to be clear?

Client: Yes.

ML: Very good. Separating those two parts completely and distinctly, so that they in no way intersect, allow yourself to go into the right hand, completely. Without any interference from the left hand, what would the right hand say about this situation?

Client: It's the situation I am in here. I have no control. It was sort of brought on by others. There is no choice. It's fairly immobile. I'm out of luck.

ML: And coming over to the left hand, what would it say about this situation?

Client: Although you didn't bring it on, and you are powerless to change others, you don't have to allow it to stay there. I can will it to move. I have recourse. And I have the power to move. It is important that I do.

ML: Coming over to the right side, what does it have to say about that?

Client: It is too big to move through the system. It is powerless, yet it is willing.

ML: What does the left side say about that?

Client: I can feel that, but you aren't powerless.

ML: Can you remember a time when you were in control? When you had the power to achieve anything that you desired?

Client: Yes. I was around eight or ten years old.

ML: I want you to fully connect with that memory now. Remember the fullness of that power, that confidence. Feel it in your body, your mind, your emotions, and in your soul. Really connect with it. And, as you do so, now, I would like to ask your subconscious mind to create for you a symbol that will represent this good feeling. What is the symbol that your subconscious mind has created for you?

Client: It's a smiley face.

ML: Very good. When you hold that smiley face, what do you experience?

Client: It is like impenetrable armor. I feel invincible.

ML: Very good. I would like you to share that smiley face with the right hand now. What do you experience as you do so?

Client: The right hand feels slightly stronger, happier. Those happier situations have existed in the past. There is no reason why they can't again, in the future.

ML: Go back to when you were between eight and ten years old. What do you remember about that time?

Client: I had the smiley face then. I had those feelings.

ML: Move ahead in time, slowly, until you notice that you lose them.

Client: It's right around when I was twelve years old. I considered myself to have a happy home life. Then it dissolved. My sister becomes anorexic. My mom is dissolving more. My dad is in denial; my grandmother, who lived just blocks away, had frequent heart problems.

ML: When these events start to occur in your life, what happens to that smiley face?

Client: The mouth goes straight, or it begins to bend downwards. The yellow fades and it is covered by a blanket. It is on the shelf in the closet.

ML: Can you go and retrieve it?

Client: Yes, I pick it up. It is smiling again. It's brighter than it was. It's been waiting for me.

ML: What would you like to do with it?

Client: I put it in my stomach. It feels warm. It's good.

ML: Now that you have done that, what does the part in your right hand think or feel about that?

Client: It is glad that it found a solution to the blockage. It had hoped all along that it wouldn't sustain the blockage. It's glad that the left hand showed it the way. It's sorry that it took so long. With the smiley face in my stomach, it will melt away the ball, that mass.

ML: Allow that to happen now . . . three, two, one. How do you feel?

Client: Much lighter.

ML: Referring back to your story, your original metaphor, now that you have these new resources, what do you notice about that story this time?

Client: The situation is still sad. It was a choice my mother made. And my sister, and my father, and even my grandmother. It was impossible for me not to be sucked into their reactions. But these were decisions they made. It was my decision to have sympathy, but I have to remember that I am not them. I am me. I have to remain detached from their failings. I can be sympathetic. But I'm a different spirit, a different soul.

ML: What do you know about your decision to come into this body, into this life situation?

Client: I was given to this family—or chose it—to work on standing up for myself. There would be forces trying to suck me into their way of life. It was a test of whether I would maintain my identity or lose it. They could be strong themselves if they had willed it.

ML: What else have you learned?

Client: I don't have to have weaknesses if I choose.

ML: What types of weaknesses are they?

Client: Although I give the illusion of strength, I have shadows of doubt in my self. I must know that there is no reason for the doubt.

ML: Would you say that there is a part of you that knows that you are strong and another part of you that creates those self-doubts?

Client: Yes.

ML: Go ahead and separate those two parts, so that the part that is confident of your strength is on one hand and the part that creates the self-doubt is on the other hand. And when you have done that, which hand has the part that is strong?

Client: The left.

ML: And the part with the self-doubt is on the right?

Client: Yes.

ML: Allow yourself to go completely into the left hand, the hand that is confident of its strength. Without any interference from the other side, what does it have to say?

Client: It is ridiculous to question my strength. It may be on the shelf in my mind, but don't question it. If I don't find my strength, I'll be a lost soul. Or I'll get sucked into the ways of my family.

ML: Moving over to the right hand, what does it have to say in the issue?

Client: No one is perfect. You can't always know everything or be strong in every situation. It would be impossible to be humble.

ML: What does the left hand have to say about that?

Client: Whatever the right hand is told, it comes from the others. Those are their perceptions, their baggage, their weaknesses, and their failings.

ML: And what does the right hand have to say about that?

Client: The right hand wants to show me I don't have to be strong, that it's a burden.

ML: By wanting to show you that, by arguing for your weakness, what is it that the right hand wants for you that is positive? What is its goal for you?

Client: It wants me to know that it is OK at times to depend on others.

ML: If you could depend on others, fully, exactly the way that the right hand wants you to, then what would you have that is even more important?

Client: Flexibility.

ML: If you could be flexible, fully, exactly the way that the right hand wants you to be, then what would you have that is even more important?

Client: More strength.

ML: If you could have more strength, fully, exactly the way that the right hand wants you to, then what would you have that is even more important?

Client: Self-esteem.

ML: If you could have self-esteem, fully, exactly the way that the right hand wants you to, then what would you have that is even more important?

Client: Love, for myself and others.

ML: If you could have love, for yourself and for others, fully, exactly the way that you imagine it there now, then what would you have that is even more important?

Client: Everlasting peace—no matter what.

ML: I would like you to imagine that everlasting peace, fully. Really turn up the volume on that peace, and experience it fully throughout your body, your mind, your emotions, and your soul. And as you do so, I would like to ask your subconscious mind to provide for you a symbol that represents this wonderful feeling. A symbol that will connect you with this feeling, each and every time that you think of it.

Client: It is a pond with gentle ripples.

ML: If you were to carry that pond and ripples with you, and this good feeling of everlasting peace, into each and every moment in the future, how would that change your experience of love of self and others?

Client: No matter what anyone else did, it would be OK. There is no reason to condemn them, but I won't lose my self-love.

ML: If you were to carry that pond and ripples with you, and this good feeling of everlasting peace, into each and every moment in the future, how would that change your experience of self-esteem?

Client: The peace allows for flexibility. It would be so peaceful that it is impossible for anyone to ruin it.

ML: If you were to carry that pond and ripples with you, and this good feeling of everlasting peace, into each and every moment in the future, how would that change your experience of being strong?

Client: I could allow myself to lean on others without chipping away my own strength. I would be adding rather than losing. I don't need to have the answers for everything.

ML: If you were to carry that pond and ripples with you, and this good feeling of everlasting peace, into each and every moment in the future, how would that change your experience of flexibility?

Client: Even when there is a give and take, it wouldn't do harm to my psyche or physical body.

ML: If you were to carry that pond and ripples with you, and this good feeling of everlasting peace, into each and every moment in the future, how would that change your experience of depending on others?

Client: It would be OK to depend on others in areas that I don't know about. That doesn't make me weaker. I'm using my resources to my advantage. I could allow access and allow their help. For my greatest good.

ML: Going back to the right hand, now, what is its perspective about all of this now?

Client: It is at peace. It is ready to make a shift.

ML: Are the right and left hands ready to work together now?

Client: Yes.

ML: Is there any part that would disagree?

Client: No.

The parts are directed to make their agreement, and we complete the integration process, as has been demonstrated in other examples. Although many techniques were involved, the entire session was completed within one hour. Notice that various techniques were incorporated within the Parts Therapy. It is important to remember to return to the parts for integration and closure before terminating the session.

CHAPTER 46

Case #9: Frank

Presenting Issues: Sports performance, inconsistency

Strategies: Regression, Empowerment Symbol, Visualization, Circle of Excellence, Parts Therapy, Outcomes, Analytical Imp, Regression, Role Model, Submodalities

Frank wanted to improve his golf game. He had been playing for many years, recreationally, and felt he should be scoring lower than he was lately. Since every golfer's problem is unique to their skill set, experience, and self-talk, discovering Frank's perspectives was the first target of our session.

ML: What do you consider to be the problem with your golf game?

Client: I am inconsistent when I am making a shot. I have trouble allowing myself to succeed. I get distracted when we are walking between holes. When I focus properly, I can shoot straight to the hole.

ML: Close your eyes and relax. Take me back to a time when you made the perfect shot. Tell me what you notice about that event.

Client: The ball leaves the club. It is a narrow fairway. The ball goes 260 yards, right down the middle.

ML: How does that make you feel?

Client: It is a feeling of success.

ML: Go back to just before the beginning of that event. Tell me what else you remember about it.

Client: I am focused on where the ball will be going. There is a sense of calm and confidence. I already know it will be good. I'm relaxed.

ML: What else do you notice?

Client: As I "pull the trigger," I am thinking, "This is so easy." It is a relaxed intensity. Like Zen.

ML: If you were to rate the intensity of that relaxation on a scale from one to ten, with ten being the most intense, what would it be?

Client: About a six.

ML: Really connect with that feeling right now, and turn up the volume. Bring it up to an eight. How does that feel?

Client: Comfortable.

ML: Now perform that same shot. What do you notice about that now?

Client: It gives a peak response.

ML: I would like to ask your subconscious mind to provide for you a symbol that will represent this good feeling of relaxation and calm. What symbol do you notice?

Client: It is a Z—a Z for "Zen"—on top of the ball.

ML: Each time you approach a golf ball, you will be able to imagine that Z right there on top, reminding you to relax this deeply. Now I wonder if you can imagine playing golf. Go to the tee and tell me what you notice.

Client: I am standing behind the ball. I look down the fairway. I see the flight of the ball in my mind. I practice swinging and then line up with the ball. I settle down, focus, and then let it flow.

ML: How does that feel?

Client: I have a sense of confidence, well-being, and calm.

ML: How was your shot?

Client: Right down the middle.

ML: Then what happens?

Client: We start walking down the fairway. We are all talking and joking around. I start to get distracted. I'm losing my focus.

ML: Imagine that there is a ten-foot diameter of protection around your ball. Each time you approach the ball, you step into the atmosphere of protection. You can leave stress, distraction, and self-doubt behind as you step into that sphere of protection. Within the sphere, there is relaxation, focused attention, and confidence. Now, walk up to the ball. What do you notice?

Client: I get into the sphere and I hit the ball 200 yards. It feels good.

ML: Then what do you notice?

Client: The ball is twenty feet from the cup. I step into the sphere, focus, and make the putt. It's a birdie. Good!

ML: Go ahead and step up to the next tee. As you are standing there, would you say that it is true that there is a part of you that knows that you can make the perfect shot and another part of you that has self-doubt?

Client: Yes.

ML: Please separate those two parts, so that the part that knows that you can make this shot is on one of your hands and the part that has self-doubt is on the other hand. Which hand knows that it can make this shot perfectly?

Client: The right hand.

ML: And the left hand has the part that has self-doubt?

Client: Yes.

ML: Separating those two parts completely and clearly, go ahead and get entirely into the right hand. Without any interference from the left hand, what does the right hand have to say about this issue?

Client: I'm confident. I can do it. I've done it before.

ML: Moving over to the left hand, what does it have to say about this?

Client: Keep the left arm straight. Balance. Twist . . . blah, blah, blah. But I don't think you can do it all the time. You're stupid. You need me to remind you. I told you so.

ML: Moving back over to the right hand, what does it have to say about what it just heard?

Client: I know how to do it. Go away and let me flow. It's easy. Consistency is letting it flow. I don't have to think too much.

ML: Moving back over to the left side, what does it have to say in response?

Client: Last time you bent your left elbow . . . blah, blah. You blew that shot.

ML: Going back to the right side, what does it have to say?

Client: If you would shut up I would do just fine. It's OK to mouth off on the practice range, but be quiet on the course.

ML: And what does the left side say about that?

Client: But you still don't turn your body enough. I need to remind you how bad you are.

ML: In doing that, what goal do you hope to achieve?

Client: To win. It thinks it needs to tell me what to do all the time.

ML: If it were able to win, all the time, fully the way that it wants to, then what would it have that is even more important?

Client: It could dominate.

ML: If it were able to dominate, fully, the way that it wants to, then what would it have that is even more important?

Client: It would be satisfied that it is fulfilled.

ML: If it were satisfied and fulfilled, fully, the way that it wants to be, then what would it have that is even more important?

Client: It would have control of my brain.

ML: If it had control of your brain, fully, the way that it wants to, then what would it have that is even more important?

Client: There is nothing more important. It could do what it wants.

ML: I am wondering if that part of your brain that is being represented as the left side would be interested in having a job that is even more important—a job that may result in an even better game of golf. What does it say?

Client: It's listening.

ML: I am wondering if it would give you its advice, and then step aside and let the other part of you, the part that wants to be in the flow with the shot, take the shot. This part could analyze, control, manipulate, and direct, and when it is time to take the shot, it can step aside and observe. Then it would have even more information to analyze, providing even better advice for you. What does it say to that?

Client: It thinks it is a good idea.

ML: What does the right hand say to this?

Client: It agrees. It has been hoping for this a long time. We also have to talk about the use of the language. The left side always gives directions and commands. We need to turn them to commentary. He needs to be polite.

ML: OK. Let's see what happens as you take the next swing. What is going on?

Client: The left hand is quiet.

ML: And the right hand?

Client: It's paying attention to the Z on the ball. It is feeling confident and balanced. It takes the shot. It's perfect.

ML: What does the left hand say?

Client: Well done. It needs recognition.

ML: How can it receive recognition?

Client: The right is confident and relaxed. In the flow. It has the right feel. The right gives the left an award. It's ego gratifying.

ML: How old does the right side feel?

Client: It feels thirty-eight years old.

ML: And the left?

Client: It feels fifty.

ML: How can you balance those ages?

Client: The thirty-eight-year-old grows up to be fifty—and that feels fine. They can be respectful friends.

ML: What does the left side say?

Client: I trust you. You know what to do. Do it!

ML: And what does the right side say?

Client: I'm in a state of relaxed intensity, focus. I'm in balance with myself and the world. I take a good shot—middle of the fairway.

ML: What does the left side say?

Client: Here we are. You know what to do. Good luck. You'll do fine.

ML: And the right?

Client: Thanks. I step into the sphere of protection. I see the Z. I close the door to distractions. Focus on the intensity and the ball. It lands on the green.

ML: And the left?

Client: The ball is fifteen feet from the hole. The pin is high, level. It's a piece of cake. I'll be quiet now. You take over.

ML: And the right?

Client: Got it! In the cup!

ML: Go to the next tee. What happens?

Client: This is the most beautiful hole on the course. My left side says, "You know what to do. I'll be quiet."

ML: What happens?

Client: I step into the zone, close the door, get the feel. My left hand started to say, "Don't screw up." We talk about that. He noticed I get tense and negative, and he doesn't want that. He changes it to, "Way to go!"

ML: Then what happens?

Client: I'm in the zone. I shoot it to the green. The left side is quiet. Then it says, "I trust you. Take over." The ball goes in the hole.

ML: Do you have a role model for golf? Is there someone you would like to emulate?

Client: Yes. David Duval.

ML: I would like you to imagine him there in front of you now. What do you notice about him?

Client: He's relaxed, confident. He stays focused, not distracted. He plays consistently.

ML: As I count from three to one, imagine stepping into his body, so that you are looking out through his eyes. Your hands are in his hands, and your feet are in his feet. Three, two, one. What do you notice about that experience?

Client: It feels good. I'm confident.

ML: Imagine teeing up and taking a shot, inside his body. What is that experience like for you?

Client: It's smooth. It feels good. I have total confidence and focus. I'm relaxed.

ML: Step up to the next shot. What do you experience?

Client: The same thing. I'm confident, focused, and relaxed. I make the perfect shot. It goes to the green. I step up to the ball and sink it in the hole.

ML: As I count from three to one, step back into your own body. Three, two, one. What do you notice about that?

Client: I'm less confident. I am more distracted. Not as sure of myself.

ML: Stepping back in . . . three, two, one. What do you notice this time?

Client: It's so easy to make a good shot. He doesn't hear the distracting voices, the comments. He can tune that out.

ML: Take the shot. What do you notice?

Client: It goes straight down the fairway. Long. It's perfect. It feels good. I'm confident.

ML: What do you notice as the fundamental differences between you and David Duval?

Client: He is self-assured, confident. He plays a consistent game. He doesn't get distracted. It feels solid in here.

ML: Do you find it interesting that you can feel that same way, yet still actually be in your own body physically? You can feel that good just by imagining it. What do you think it might be like if you were to step into David Duval's energy field each time you make a shot?

Client: That would be great. I would be consistent, sure of myself, focused.

ML: Imagine that each time you approach a ball in the future, you step into that sphere of protection, shedding the old ways and taking on the David Duval frame of mind. Each time you approach the ball, you notice the *Z* for Zen, in your mind's eye. You get in the zone, and consistently shoot with a focused, confident mindset. What do you think that will be like?

Client: It feels great!

This session was brought to a close with a few suggestions to remember everything learned and experienced during the session. Notice that we used a modification of the Circle of Excellence technique to provide protection from distraction. Frank later reported that the next time he played golf, his score was seventeen points lower than his previous average game. He was thrilled!

It is a recognized fact, in sports, that the mind game is as important as the physical practice. Helping clients in sports performance is a growing and lucrative field.

Bibliography

Andreas, Connirae, and Steve Andreas. *Heart of the Mind.* Moab, Utah: Real People Press, 1989.

Andreas, Connirae, and Tamara Andreas. *Core Transformation: Reaching the Wellspring Within.* Moab, Utah: Real People Press, 1994.

Bandler, Richard, and John Grinder. *Frogs into Princes: Neuro-Linguistic Programming.* Moab, Utah: Real People Press, 1979.

——. *Reframing: Neuro-Linguistic Programming and the Transformation of Meaning.* Moab, Utah: Real People Press, 1982.

Brandon, Nathaniel. *The Six Pillars of Self-esteem.* New York: Bantam Books, 1994.

Chopra, Deepak. *Quantum Healing: Exploring the Frontiers of Mind/Body Medicine.* New York: Bantam Books, 1989.

de Bono, Edward. *de Bono's Thinking Course.* Rev. ed. New York: Facts on File, 1994.

Durbin, Paul G. *Kissing Frogs: The Practical Uses of Hypnotherapy.* Dubuque, Iowa: Kendall/Hunt, 1996.

Elias, Jack. *Finding True Magic: A Radical Synthesis of Eastern and Western Perspectives and Techniques.* Seattle: Five Wisdoms, 1999.

Gibson, H. B. *Hypnosis: Its Nature and Therapeutic Uses.* New York: Taplinger, 1977.

Grinder, John, and Richard Bandler. *The Structure of Magic.* Vol. 1 and 2. Moab, Utah: Real People Press, 1975, 1976.

——. *Trance-Formations: Neuro-Linguistic Programming and the Structure of Hypnosis.* Moab, Utah: Real People Press, 1981.

Hogan, Kevin. *The New Hypnotherapy Handbook: Hypnosis and Mindbody Healing.* Kearney, Nebr.: Morris, 2001.

Hogan, Kevin, and Mary Lee LaBay. *Through the Open Door: Secrets of Self-Hypnosis.* Gretna, La.: Pelican, 2000.

Lucas, Winafred Blake. *Regression Therapy: A Handbook for Professionals.* Vol. 1 and 2. Crest Park, Calif.: Deep Forest, 1999.

Mader, Sylvia. *Understanding Human Anatomy and Physiology.* Dubuque, Iowa: Times Mirror Higher Education Group, 1997.

Philips, George, and Terence Watts. *Rapid Cognitive Therapy: The Professional Therapist's Guide to Rapid Change Work.* Vol. 1. Carpathian, Wales: Crown House, 1999.

Phillips, Maggie, and Claire Frederick. *Healing the Divided Self: Clinical and Ericksonian Hypnotherapy for Post Traumatic and Dissociative Conditions.* New York: Norton, 1995.

Rosen, Sidney. *My Voice Will Go With You: The Teaching Tales of Milton H. Erickson.* New York: Norton, 1991.

Rossi, Ernest Lawrence. *The Psychobiology of Mind-Body Healing: New Concepts of Therapeutic Hypnosis.* New York: Norton, 1986.

Rubin, Zick, Letitia Anne Peplau, and Peter Salovey. *Psychology.* Boston: Houghton Mifflin, 1993.

Index

For more information about
Mary Lee LaBay
you are invited to visit
www.maryleelabay.com